Why Own a Dog:

The Incredible

Captain Buddy

How to
Convince
Someone
Into
Buying a Dog

Kathleen Nansel Rogers

Dedicated

to
Captain Buddy,
and for all other
Dog Owners.
May they stay in our hearts forever!

We are all guided by a beating heart.
Life is the game made for everyone,
and Love is the prize.
Unconditional Love,
The ultimate of all Love,
Other than God,
A dog enables you to feel their
soft coat, hug them, converse with them
and interact with one of Gods
Creations, in the best way ever!
You will realize that you didn't know that
you were lost,
until you've owned
a
Dog.

All photographs
by
Kathleen Nansel Rogers

CONTENTS

Part One:

The

True Story

Of a

Soft Coated Wheaton Terrier

Captain
Buddy

(Born February 21, 2004

- February 29, 2020)

Acknowledgements

My heartfelt thanks go to all the dogs, and
dog owners, that Captain Buddy and I
encountered
along the many adventurous journeys
together.
Through Buddy, I learned that other people
are us greatest resource – through that of
owning a dog.

1

How to Convince Dad to Get a Dog

Get in the truck!

Where are we going?

We're going to get a dog for Loren.

I got a huge smile on my face!

For years Richard has said that he didn't

want a dog or a cat.

Even when I first moved in with him, he had

me get rid of my cat, and I just previously had

to put my dog down. For years since we had

our daughter Loren, he has said no to getting

a dog.

I think that I know what got him to

change his mind.

One day while I was jogging in the Little Big

Econ State Forest, about 10,000 acres, near

our home, after a forest control burning, I

discovered a baby turtle that had been

seriously burned. It was so small that I could

hold it in my hand closed and you would not

be able to see it. I brought it home and

carefully cleaned it using a soft toothbrush.

I showed it to Loren, and it became her only pet. She named it Emma and Emma went everywhere with Loren. She even brought her to the New Millennium Mall, in her baby doll stroller, all decked out with many other dolls and everything you would possibly need as well as in its proper place. It was a real jaw dropper when salespeople and total strangers would be observing her of being so meticulous in picking up her dolls one at a time to attend to their needs with various items and then, they would give a special attention, when she would turn around, and pick up her turtle Emma!

Every morning she would place Emma on the kitchen table as she ate her bowl of Cream of Wheat, and would put a scoop on the table, so that Emma could eat breakfast with her, before going to school. It was so cute to see this turtle, a reptile, express a personality of its own, even just by the way it cocked its head, looking up at you and then carefully brought out its tongue, to scoop up the Cream of Wheat, and close its eyes as if to express how good it tasted.

<u>She became very close to this turtle, her only pet.</u>

One day, when I came home from work, she showed me that her Dad made a corral for Emma. It was a shiny rich white painted wood with nice brand-new gold hinges, so that she could create a corral anywhere and contain Emma. It wasn't until weeks later that I discovered my very first painting easel, from when I was ten years old, made of rich black walnut was missing! He had cut up my easel for Emma's corral!

Oh well, Loren is happy to have a pet and so am I.

Then one day, I found myself stopping short in my step, when I heard Richard talking sweet and comforting to someone outside.

To my surprise, that someone, was Emma!

 He was holding her gently in his hands and talking to her.

Then one day, Emma was missing! She had either gotten out of the pool area and could not be found. This really upset Loren!

2

Buying a Dog

So here we are at a Pet Store, looking at cute lively puppy dogs!

Look at that cute white curly one.

Oh, his fur is so soft!

What is he?

A <u>Soft - Coated Wheaton Terrier.</u>

As I read from a chart that the pet shop had

hanging in the store.

They are hypoallergenic, meaning that
they don't shed their coat.

Temperament: Affectionate,

Intelligent, Energetic, Spirited, Playful,
and Faithful.

They were bred in Ireland, bred for
herding sheep, catching varmints on
the farm, and they like to go for long
walks in the woods.

That's me I thought!

They are very loving without being
clingy because they also love their
independence.

This was so true.

Buddy was affectionate, but he wasn't
always needing attention, like some
dog breeds.

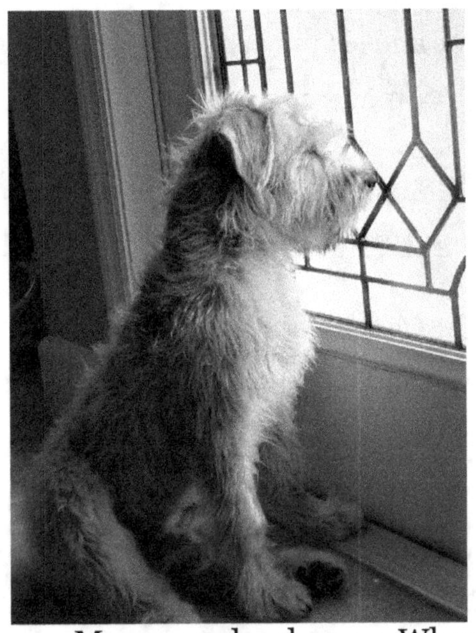

Many people who own Wheaton

Terriers, name them Radar, because
they are gatherers, always going
throughout the house making sure that
everyone is accounted for, and when
one member of the family is gone they

will be devoted to waiting for them at

the door and sleep where that family
member sleeps.

**<u>This turned out to be so
astonishingly true!</u>**

I thought what a perfect match for our
family and happily, we brought
Captain Buddy home with us, but little
did we know the adventures and
journeys that he would take us on. Oh,
were they wonderful!

3

Captain Buddy Love's Water!

Our daughter Loren, named him Buddy, which seemed appropriate, since she was the only child still at home, but to give him royalty, I added Captain Buddy, because my husband was a Captain Airline Pilot, and my son named his West Highland Terrier,

Captain Chuckles.

It was so much fun to watch him jump
real, high in a relaxing horizontal
position over our large cool blue pool
water, with his front paws so

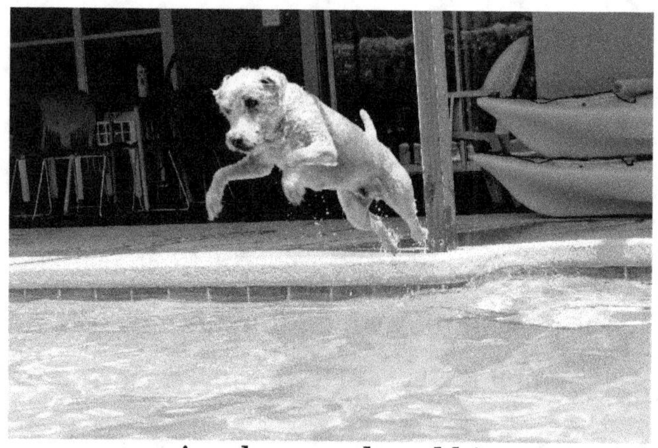

graciously curved, and his ears

vertically up in the air, expressing
dignity and strength!

Jumping after Loren, in the pool, he also
loved swimming after and chasing her for
sometimes, hours. It really put smiles on

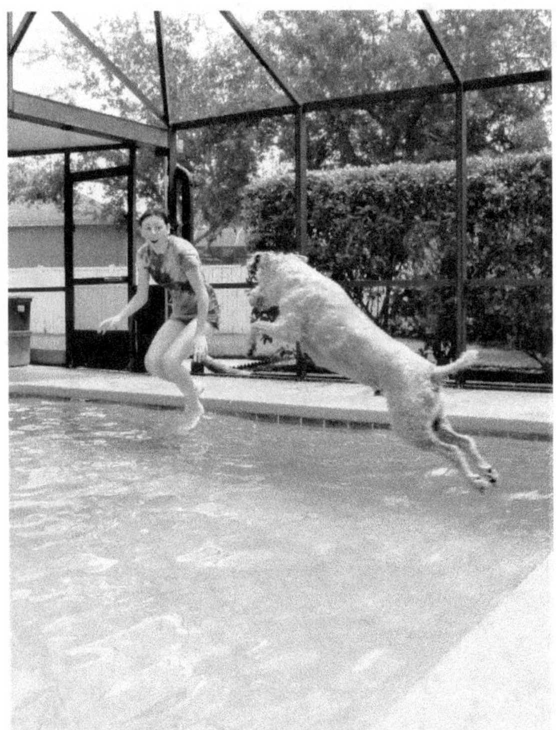

everyone's faces, to see this unexplainable

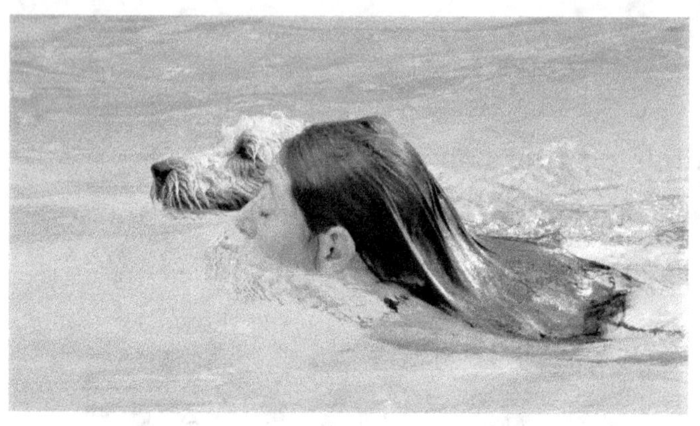

bond between them!

Loren wouldn't even have to say
anything. She would just point, or give
a quick flick in the air, with her finger
and he would follow her commands.

Loren and Buddy were such a joy to
watch swim together.

Loren later, ended up being on the

swimming team, and the water polo
team in High School, and a Bio-
Medical Degree, and a Nursing Degree.

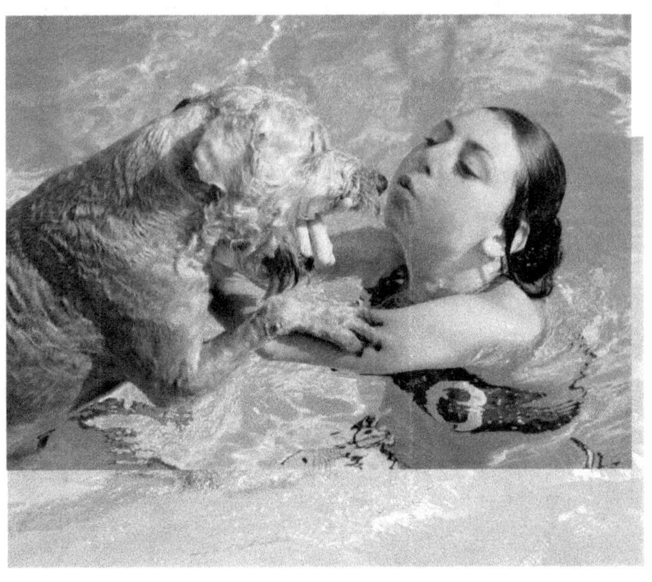

It was even more enjoyable to watch

and hear Buddy give out playful and
childish whines and humorous out
cries when Loren would gently give
playful gestures of covering his eyes
and quickly moving her hand away, or

gently blowing into his ear, while he
would be in the pool or standing above
her at the 'poolside and she in the
water.

Buddy also was the shark in the pool
chasing all of Loren's friends, with as
many as ten kids at the same time! It
was surprising to see all of them run
out of energy and would have to resort
to getting out of the pool before him to
rest! Buddy was the life of the party.
Every time!

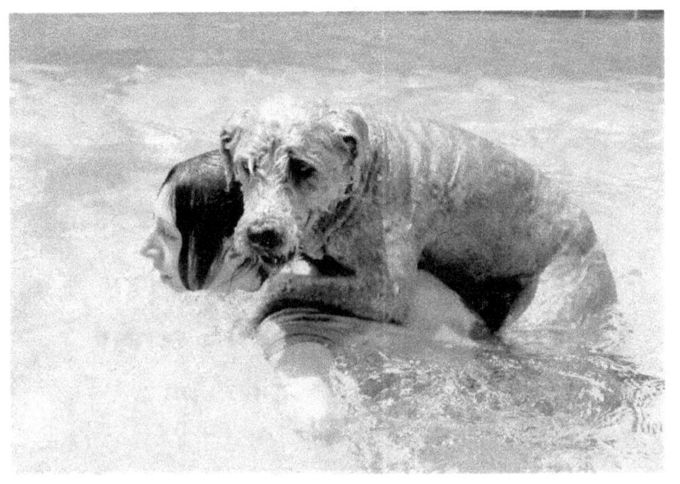

He loved to ride on Loren's back in the
pool and with a look of such content,
he made it appear that he could stay on
her back for ever.

Buddy could stay in the water for hours.

I have never seen another dog that could keep up with Buddy.

I have watched him play with many different dog breeds, and even the top water dog breeds, such as Labrador Retrievers, and Golden Retrievers in every environment, and in many different places, such as in the Econ river, Riverside Park river, Atlantic Ocean, other Lakes, Maine, and our

20 x 40-foot swimming pool.

Some of these breeds, would only be interested in their owner, who was throwing a ball in the water. This would aggravate Buddy, because he

could see after a while that they
weren't playing with him!

He's played with Wheaton's, and
Poodles, in the water, but they only
would stay for a matter of minutes.

4

Dog Parks

I remember the first time that Buddy went into the water. It was at Lake Baldwin Dog Park, in Winter Park, Florida. What a neat place to visit, even if you don't own a dog. On any given weekend, you could see about a

hundred different dog breeds at this park running in the wooded area and swimming in the lake, with its soft white sandy beach.

At one stage of his life, I would take
him there almost every weekend.

My first time arriving there, they told
me that you must let him off his leash,
because the other dogs will attack him.

I was at first hesitant, because Terriers
will give a protective approach, and
other dogs might think that he is being
mean, but that is just a Terrier's
approach, to being friendly.

So, I released him from his leash, and

someone came up to talk to me and
then I lost track of Buddy.

I then, heard a woman say, look at that
dog swimming under water! Low and
behold, it was Buddy, swimming
completely under water!

He never ceased to amaze me! This was his first, time swimming in the water. He got so excited chasing with a group of Golden Retrievers, who were always going after a ball into the lake.

I then started to get discouraged in going to the Dog Parks, because Buddy kept getting attacked by other dogs. I didn't discover why Buddy was all most always being attacked at the dog park until his vet told me that it is because he was not fixed and the other dogs at the park knew that he had something they did not, and they wanted it. So that explains why there were fights.

The first time that it happened was when he got into a fight with a

German Sheppard! Buddy made the
big full-grown bad looking dog squeal!
Everyone at the park laughed when I
heard a woman say,

"And he's so soft and fluffy too!"

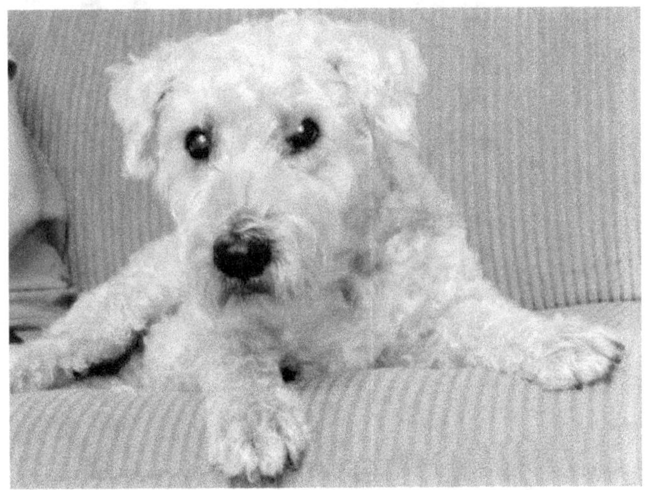

5

First Time in The

Forest

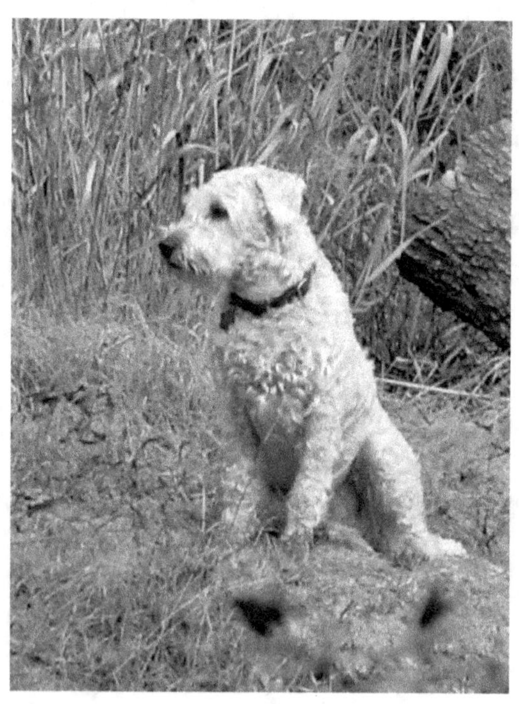

Another stage of Buddy's life, for years on weekends I would take him in the Little Big Econlockhatchee State Forest, about 10,000 acres of woods, only across the street from our home, 6 minutes while sitting on my bike seat.

This forest is part of the Florida National Scenic Trail, about 2,000 miles long, going from the Florida Panhandle, all the way to south of Miami, Bald Cypress Lake.

This section is one of the most beautiful trails, going along the Little Big Econlockatchee River.

There are five trailheads into this gorgeous forest.

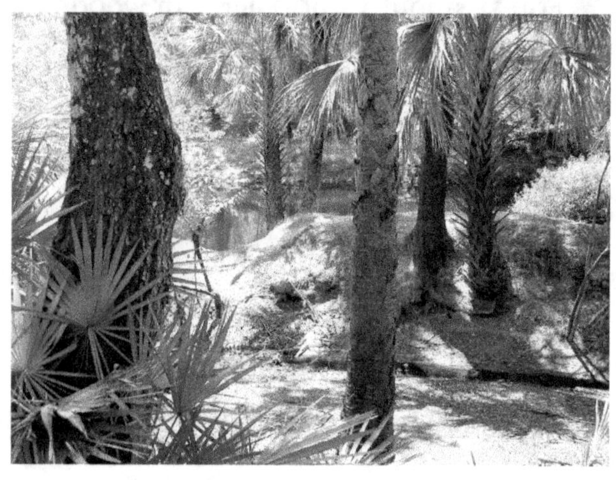

Each trailhead is designated for different activities. There is the Jones Trailhead, which is for Mountain Biking, The Equestrian Trailhead, for horseback riding, The Flagler Trailhead, for biking and hiking. The Kolokee Loop Trailhead, for hiking, which I also liked for a while, because Buddy and I would always see a lot of wildlife on this trail, and

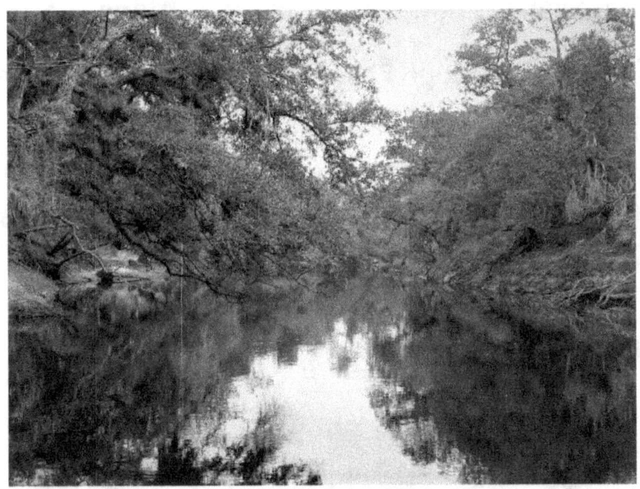

The Barr Street Trailhead is the only one that

is along the river, (17 miles through the forest
and empties into the St. Johns River) strictly
hiking and is part of the National Scenic Trail
(only 7 in the USA. that are 1,000 miles or
more). This is the trailhead, that we ventured
on the most together.

On the Barr Street Trailhead, the Florida National Scenic Trail, which takes you along the scenic river, and over seven quaint wooden bridges, over inviting tributaries. Each bridge offers different viewpoints of the river, a variety of plant life, and terrain.

For example, going over the first one, are mostly large Live Oak trees, the second one, takes you through luscious palm trees, with white powdery sandy path, the third one takes you overlooking the river from above eye

level, the fourth bridge, is in the
deepest part of the forest, (the
quietest), which most surely you will

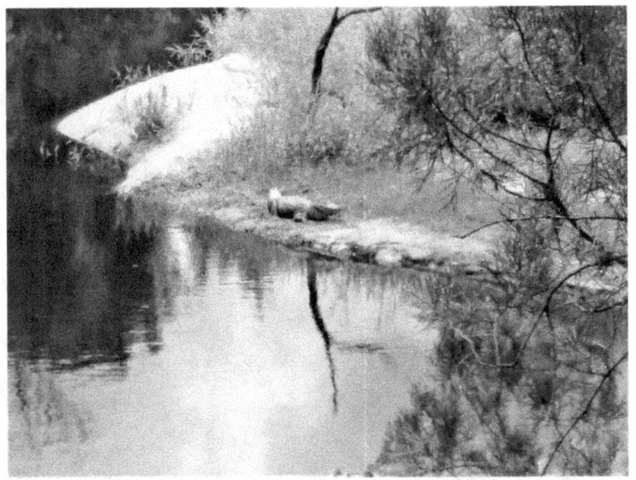

witness an alligator basking on the

white sandy embankment, on the opposite
side of the river, the fifth bridge gives you
more likelihood of seeing an owl, so keep your
eyes peeled at the treetops, and

the sixth bridge, gives you a glimpse of
the seventh bridge, the largest, that

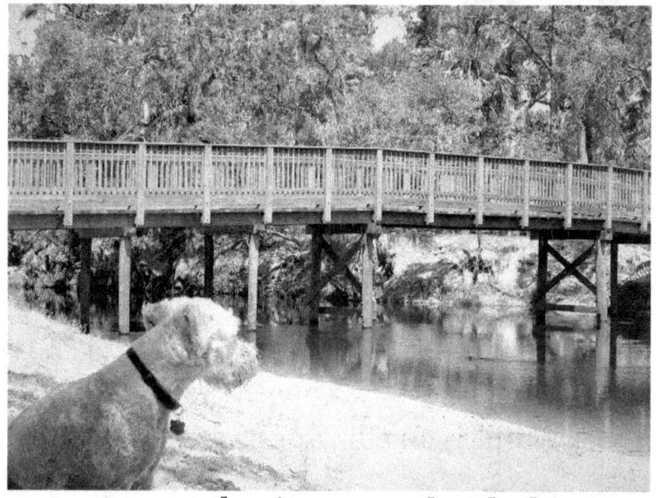

goes across the river, onto the Flagler

Trail. Buddy and I have met many
interesting people and have had many
different animal encounters
throughout the 20 years exploring this

gorgeous forest.

One time we met a young lady, who was a U.C.F. college student, who said that she couldn't afford to go to school that summer, or pay for her room and board, so, she said that she was going to hike the Florida National Trail, for the summer. You can go along this trail and camp. She said that she had a friend drop her off 23 miles south of where we were, and she wanted to know if there was a grocery store nearby. After giving her directions, I asked her if she was doing the trail all by herself, and she said, just me and my pistol! After she showed me her gun, I asked her how much her backpack weighed about.

She said that it was about 30 pounds,

because your hiking pack should not

weigh more than about 10% of your
body weight. I wished her good luck
and Buddy and I continued the trail.

One time on the Kolokee Loop Trail,
Buddy and I stopped in our tracks,
because we thought that we heard a

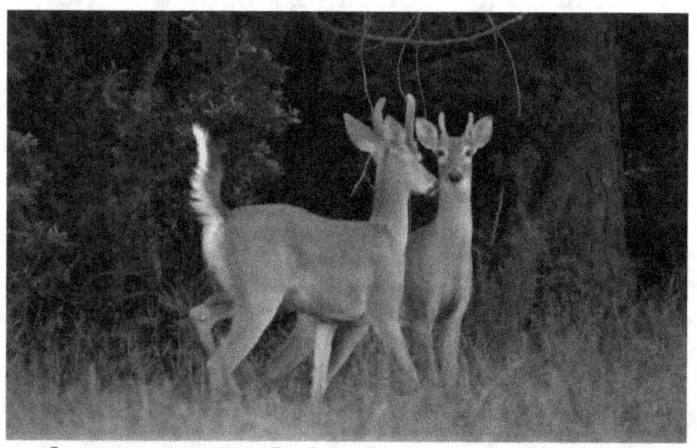

horse running behind us! It turned out
to be a huge Buck!

I then came upon an elderly man fishing, and he told me that this deer has been in these woods for about 20 years.

I guess this Buck was wise enough to stay in an area that there was no hunting allowed. Buddy was with me almost every weekend, doing many things for hours each time in this gorgeous forest.

Such as Plein - air painting, (to capture a sense of a place with color oil and light, painting with my oil bars), kayaking, biking, sketching, sunbathing, exploring, hiking, swimming, horseback riding, creating pirate treasure maps for my art students, and just hanging out on the riverbank, taking in natures wonder and wildlife.

I will never forget the first time that I took Buddy in this forest. It was in the Econ and we were sitting on the white sandy ground overlooking the river to take in the surroundings, and I was observing Buddy's reaction.

Suddenly, we heard a Great Horn Owl make a loud; Who, Who, Who, Whooooo! "Who cooks for you, who cooks for you all?

"I watched Buddy's eyes turn sideways
first, while sitting straight, his jaw
drop, and then his head bowing down,
and then turning ever so slowly to
scope out the treetops, with an

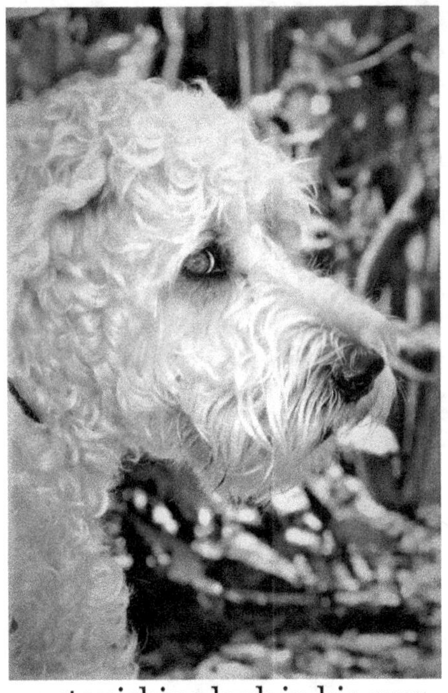

astonishing look in his eyes.

You could tell that this was his first time experiencing the forest. He loved it!

Now that I reflect on it, this spot where he first experienced the forest, was always his favorite spot, which you had to go over 7 bridges, about 5.2mile trail loop, to go to this location.

6

Many Adventures in The Forests

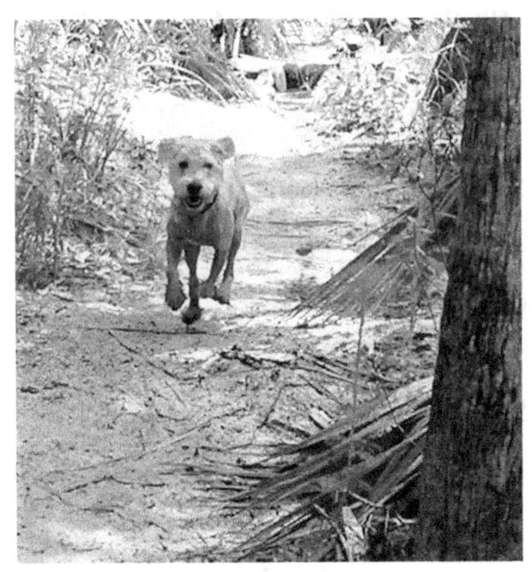

One time after the many times that
Buddy ran alongside me while I
mountain biked through the many
winding forest trails, dodging trees,
roots, dips, and flying up high, going
down through creeks, and over a
variety of terrain such as white sandy
paths, autumn leaves, or pine nettles,
nestled on the ground to wet swampy
areas of light green moss, and the
many different environmental settings,
from tall wispy pine trees to open soft
grassy pastures, surrounded by
hundred-year-old Live Oak Trees, saw
palmetto's, a wide-open field of acres
filled with yellow, orange flowers, (the
Florida State yellow tick seed flower),

and a forest of nothing but majestic
palm trees.

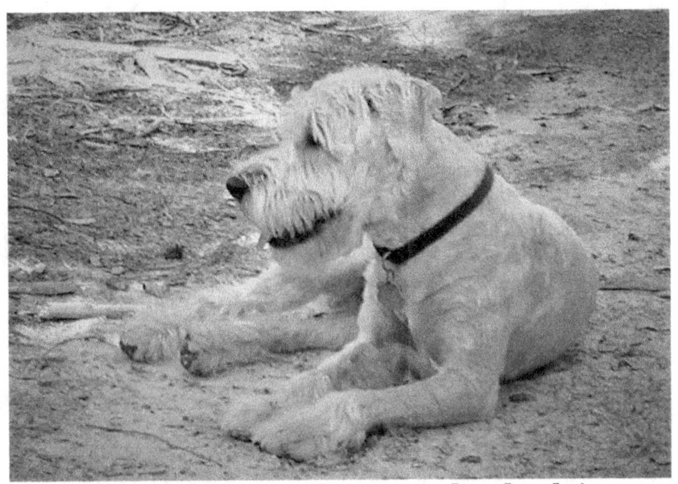

I laid down on the ground to bask in
the sun, only to be woken by Buddy
grabbing a guy's ankle as he quietly
road his mountain bike by me. I could
always count on Buddy, to protect me.

There were many times in the forest, that Buddy sensed someone's intentions were not good, and he growled or snipped at them.

7

Terrier Persistence

One of the things that I like about terriers is that they are not afraid of anything or anyone. They are going to stand their ground to protect you no matter what the circumstances!

I know that this is true because I have owned terriers for about 50 years. Two Scottish Terriers, Maggie & Bonnie, a West Highland Terrier, Captain Chuckles, and Captain Buddy, a Soft Coated Wheaton Terrier.

To understand a terrier's natural
instincts will help one to appreciate
and value them.

I have witnessed this time after time
their unstoppable persistence.

Another time when I was plein-air
painting and I had him tied up to a tree
by the river embankments when a pit
bull appeared.

Buddy warned him, but he attacked
Buddy and they fought while rolling
down into the river.

The owner got their dog and
apologized, but Buddy ended up losing
two teeth and some bite wounds from
trying to protect me.

Again, another time after painting for hours, in the Econ. I took Buddy down into a palm forest to take a pee. After hooking his retractable leash on a palm frond, a wild boar appeared, and Buddy bolted after him.

I watched Buddy chase him with the retractable leash flying up in the air each time that he jumped over a tree lying on the ground and my last site of him, was when he was leaping in the air about to pounce down on this huge wild boar! I walked through the forest calling and looking for Buddy for three and a half hours, through thick tall palm fronds, poisonous cotton mouth snake everywhere! It was scary.

When he finally came running to me, I noticed that he had chewed the tough

retractable leash lead completely
gone! He must have gotten tangled and
was chewing it while I was calling him.

During the month of February, is
mating season, for the Great Horn
Owl. One time late at night, with
flashlight in hand, Buddy and I
set out into the Little Big Econ State
Forest to experience the Great Horn
Owls at their most vocal time of the
year! Buddy was one incredibly brave
dog.
It was several miles in
the darkest forest ever, before we got
down to the river and sat down under
an over a hundred-year-old Live Oak
Tree, where Buddy initially
experienced the Great Horn
Owl, but tonight was different,

because there were many Great Horn
Owls whooping and were extremely
loud! It was such an awesome
moment!

Just a little trivia, looking at Buddy's
right ear in this pic, and following the
only dead tree, in the background, is
where Buddy and I have
witnessed a Kennedy Space launch,
and as we watched it go off, a Bald
Eagle, flew off this tree.

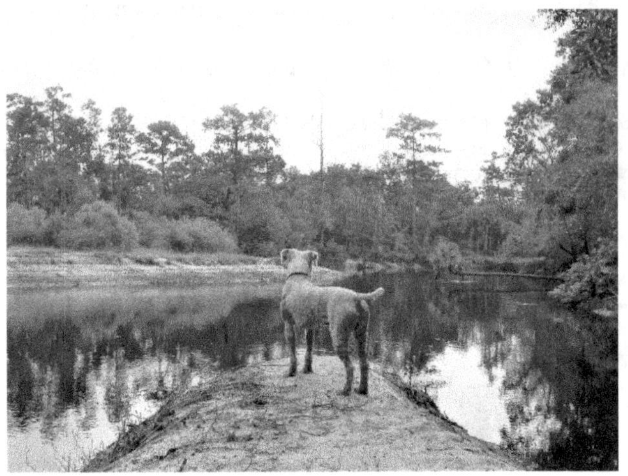

Buddy was always scoping varmints out.
 Even while we would be hiking on a trail.
There were many a time that even on his
leach, he snatched something out of its hiding
place. Armadillo, Opossum, Squirrel, Rabbit,
or a Dove.
 He was good at getting lizards too!
 He always made sure that one did not set
foot on his pool territory. Another time was at
my property, I named Clear Landing, because
of discovering a WWI, airplane propeller, in
an over hundred-year-old shed, on about 2
acres, which is nestled in 53,000 acres of
forest, some owned by the Mormons, who
 have cattle.

Buddy had escaped, was gone for
hours, when he reappeared with a herd

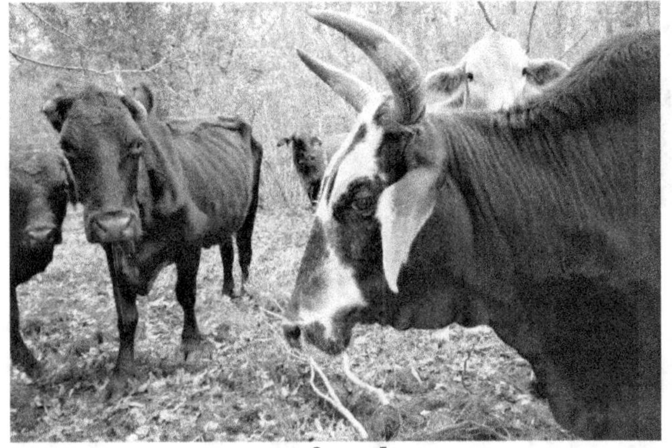

of cattle

and multiple huge bulls, who were
threatening him, charging him with their
horns and he still stood his ground barking at
them.

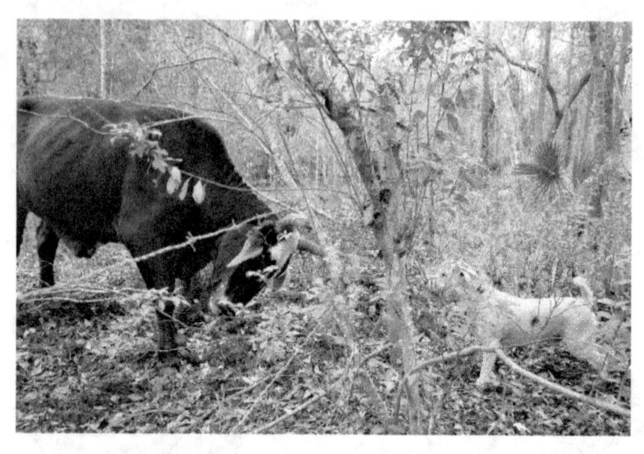

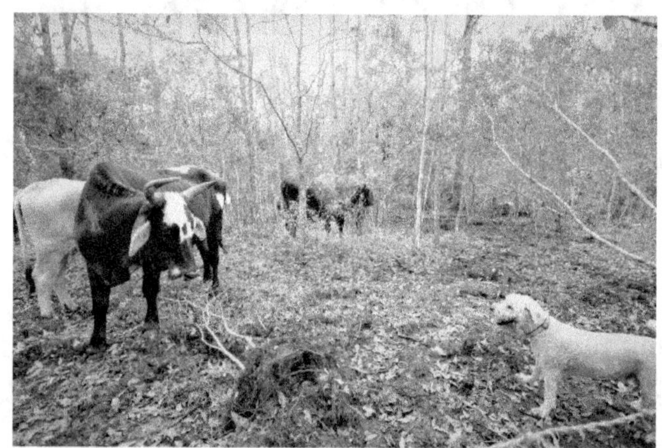

A real jaw dropper!

Another time was when a cow came up

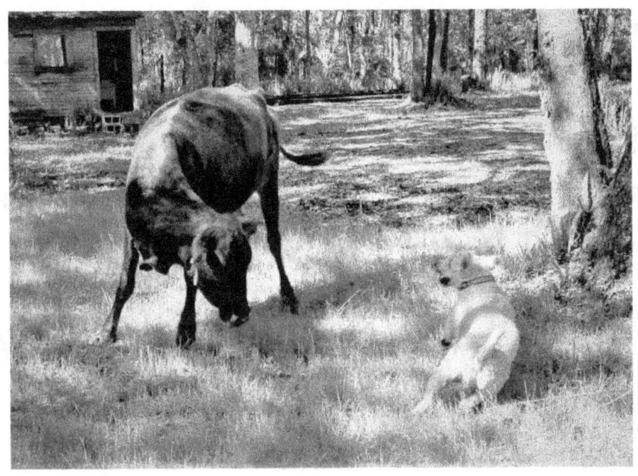

from the creek, on Clear Landing, my property to get to my luscious green grass, and Buddy was defending his territory, as usual.

Again, another time was when we were kayaking down the Little Big Econ State

Forest River, as Buddy stood at the bow of the boat, within small quarters, either in front, in the back or in between my legs for hours while going down the Econ River, there was a huge alligator on the sandy shoreline and Buddy jumped from the boat running towards it. I screamed slapping the oar on the water's surface calling him!

Luckily the alligator ignored Buddy, and just as I got him in the boat again, another Alligator's large

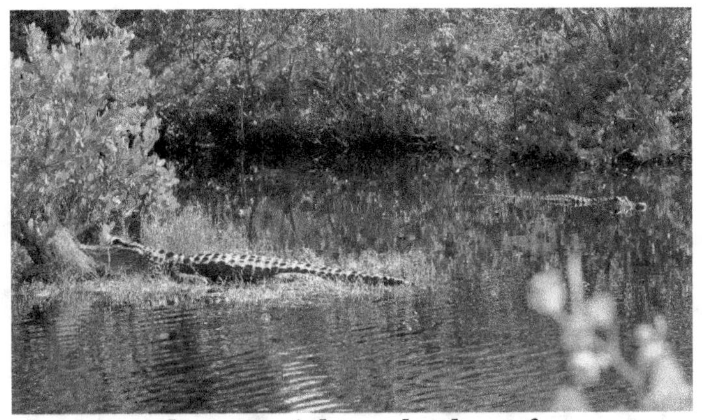

head appeared, at my right, only about four

feet away. It was intimidating, sitting low in

the kayak, with one alligator sitting up high

on the white sandy bank, and the other one
to my right in the water, where its head was
so big, that its eyes were only inches from the

top of the Kayak! I've read that for every inch

from a gator's eyes to its nose, is how long

they are in feet.

This was at the very least, a 10-footer for sure!

We even had one cross our path one time.

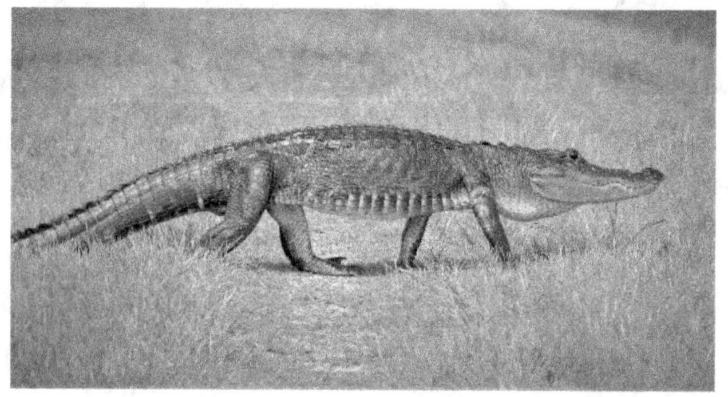

In the winter months, when the river
would be low, we would wade in it,
looking for fish and Buddy would cock
his head, moving it ever so quickly
back and forth, and when he would eye
one, he would go under the water to
catch it.

Of course, it would get away, but he
did come close to getting a fish one
time.

I did have a picture of buddy in the
front of one of my kayaks that
strangers took a picture of along the
River, but I haven't been able to find it.

Here is one on the lake in our

back yard, on Christmas Day, 2019,

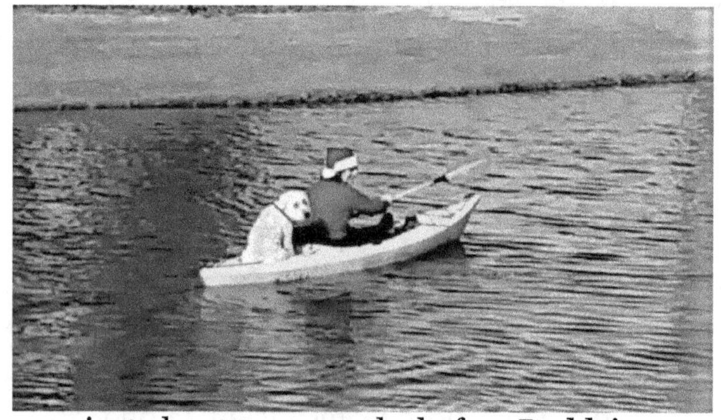

just about two months before Buddy's

death, in February. Note how devoted he was,
and us not knowing that he had a Stomach
Tumor growing, inside of him. Often when we
went kayaking down the river, Buddy would
be in the front, jump off the kayak, swim to
the other side of the river,

scope out the land by smelling around, come back to me then go to the other side. I had to make sure that he was not in stagnant water, because this is where alligators like to stay, they do not like it where the current is flowing. This was also the time that Buddy loved to swim after the river otters across the Econ and I would have to wade after him, on the other side.

Again, another time was when Buddy
and I were enjoying hours of some
quiet quality time of swimming in the
oup

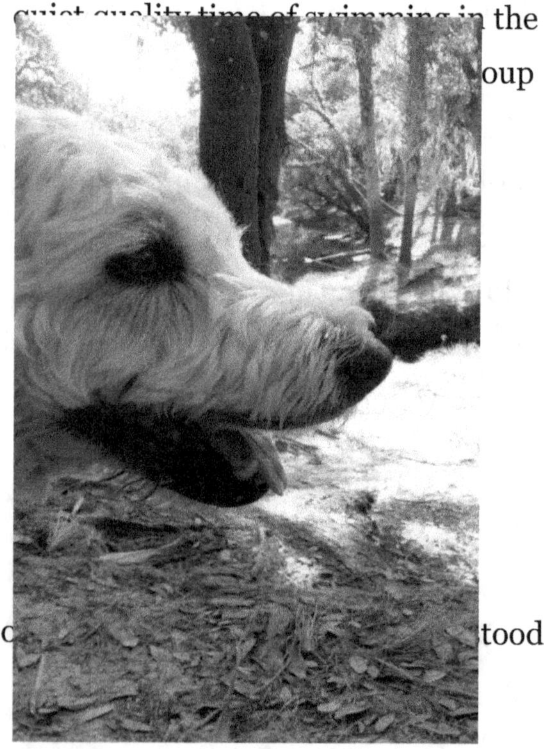

tood

his ground barking at the horses, when

suddenly, one of the horses kicked
him in the head so hard that you could
hear a loud thud sound, but that didn't
stop Buddy!

He only paused for a moment only to
continue barking until they left! From
this moment on, he did not like horses.

Another time, which reflects his breed
characteristics of catching varmints on
the farm.at Clear Landing there is an
over hundred, year old shed that
Buddy spent hours many a time trying
to scope a varmint out by even biting
at the shed wood and digging around
it.

One time I discovered him inside of it on the
very top of mostly empty plastic totes, which

was amazing that he didn't come tumbling down from them. Such persistence and determination, incredible!

Unstoppable and relentlessly Captain Buddy stood his ground even to lightning and thunder when it rained! At the sound of lightening or thunder, he would run out to the pool patio, in the rain barking and howling as all four legs would jump up in the air at the same time and coming down with a firm pounce.

It always brought a big smile followed by laughter from everyone who was fortunate to be in his presence.

8

Clear Landing

&

Homer

One time when Buddy was playing with Loren in the pool, he hurt one of his front legs. Instead of leaving him at home alone I brought him with me to the property, Clear Landing, so that I could cut the grass and he

could be surrounded by a different
environment, seeing, smelling and
hearing different sounds, and for him
to see Homer, my horse in hopes to
create a bond, between the both. This
picture is the first time that Buddy met
Homer, my horse.

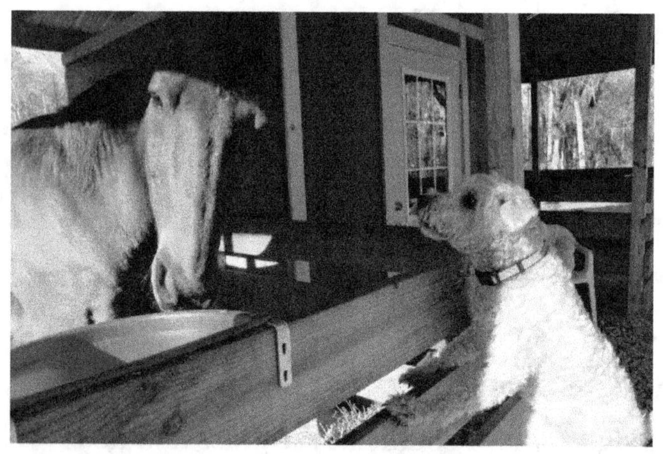

Buddy the alpha of Clear Landing, (the
first to be at the property),

a couple of years, before Homer. I tried to get Buddy to except Homer.

One time I walked them, by myself at the same time in Tosohatchee Wildlife Management Area, 33,000 acres of forest, determined to get them to accept one another. I had some close calls with them from time to time, but it never worked out. Making sure that he was on a chain lead/runner, my horse Homer, so open, giving, and excepting of any animal to come his way, went up to greet Buddy, was not aware that Buddy could reach him, and Buddy immediately got under Homers belly and started biting him. Homer quickly tried to get away, but he got tangled in Buddy's lead, and he fell on Buddy. After checking

Buddy, he seemed fine, so I tied him
up on the deck around the cabin. Later
Buddy jumped down from the deck
and then lifting his previously injured
leg up in the air and shaking it, I could
see that it was broken!

I immediately took him to his
Veterinarian, they said that they could
not do anything for him, that the leg
would have to be amputated.

The vet put a cast on any way and
after months of healing, so we thought,
but discovered that his bones were not
even connected, when the Vet removed
it. So, I then had to decide to have
surgery on the leg and have him in a
cast again and hope that it would heal
a second time!

After this second surgery, when the
Vet brought him out, I got on the floor
to hug, caressed and gave a comforting
whine. Buddy reacted by giving me the
same sound back, like he always did,
but this one was exceptionally long and
profound! The next thing that I noticed
was the receptionist was leaning over
the counter to look down at us in
astonishment and disbelief!

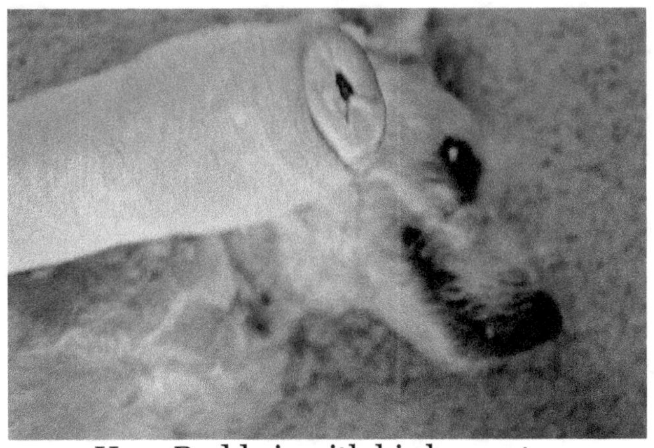

Here Buddy is with his leg cast on.

9

Halloween

I remember Buddy's first Halloween! We bought him a dog Football jersey and shorts. He got loose, went around our lake, through a new neighbor's garage, into their living room, sat down on the carpet rug in front of their huge Television screen, and was watching TV.

When the neighbor came down the stairs. He told me that at first, he didn't know what or who it was!

His shorts though are still a mystery
as to where they ended up, never to

be found.

Another Halloween was when I took
Buddy in to get him fixed. When I went
to pick him up at the Vets office in Pets
Smart, I noticed that they were having
a Dog Halloween party, a dog costume
contest, with prizes and free dog food
and treats! Remembering that Loren
and I had previously gotten Buddy a
Zorro costume, I rushed him home,
put on his costume, and he looked so
cute, with the Zorro hat and cape yet a
little bad at the same

time. As we were entering the store,
with Buddy walking slow because of
him still being sore,

we both stopped at the door because of
two large black, bad looking dogs, with
costumes that were real tight fitting
shiny and red and black, that showed
their muscles when they walked. I
remember one was a Doberman. They
looked down at Buddy and Buddy
looked up at them not only in pain but
with vulnerability and not a single
growl or sound came out of him.

He didn't win any prize, because to my
surprise, every dog in there was decked
out in gorgeous, custom fitted,
outstanding outfits!

One lady had a couple of dogs that
were dressed as Bride and Groom,
Bride in a beautiful white wedding

dress, and the Groom, a luscious Tuxedo. Their outfits were so nicely fitted and enjoyable to see; I don't remember the breed of dogs that they were. I also thought, boy what an awesome community we moved into, to have so many dog owners take such extra effort to prepare and show off their dogs.

10

Buddy Rides

He loved going for rides in the red and
green child carrier attached to my bike.
I took him in the Econ State Forest in it,
explored other towns, trails, Publix
grocery store and at least once a week in
and around our huge, thousand home
Oviedo, subdivision, called

Live Oak Reserve.

He was such a trooper!

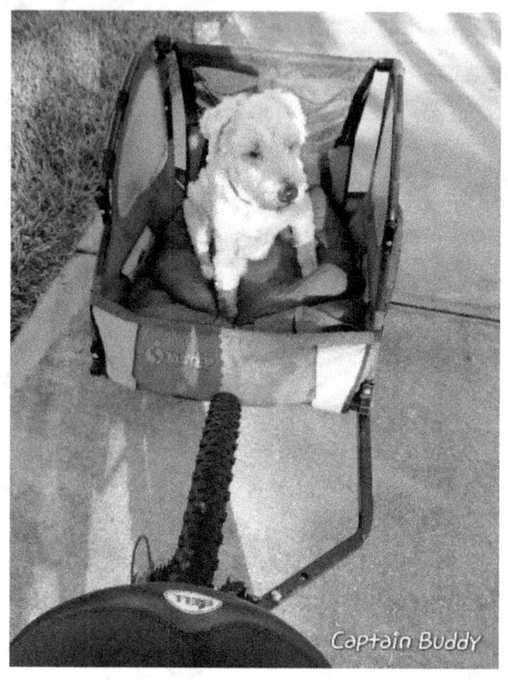

Everyone we ever met couldn't believe
how well behaved he was every place that we
took him. Even on the carts sometimes for
hours at Lowe's or Home Depot as we decided

on the many items to buy.

Buddy would even stay on Loren's
narrow motorized scooter as she rode him

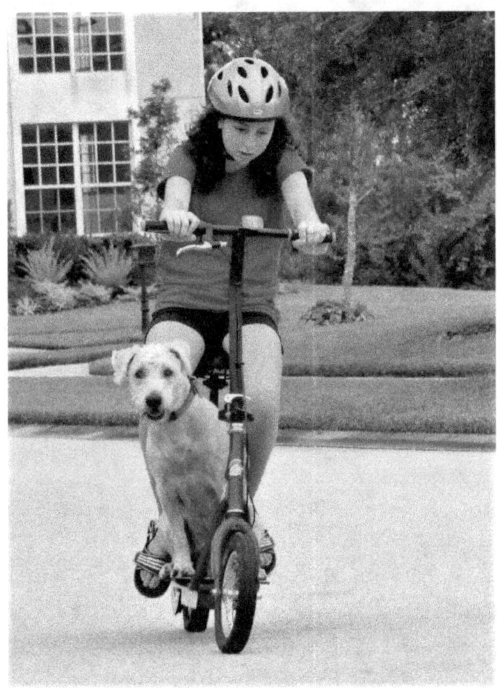

around the subdivision. He would

sit content and looked confident, in an
exploring mode, without a worry in the

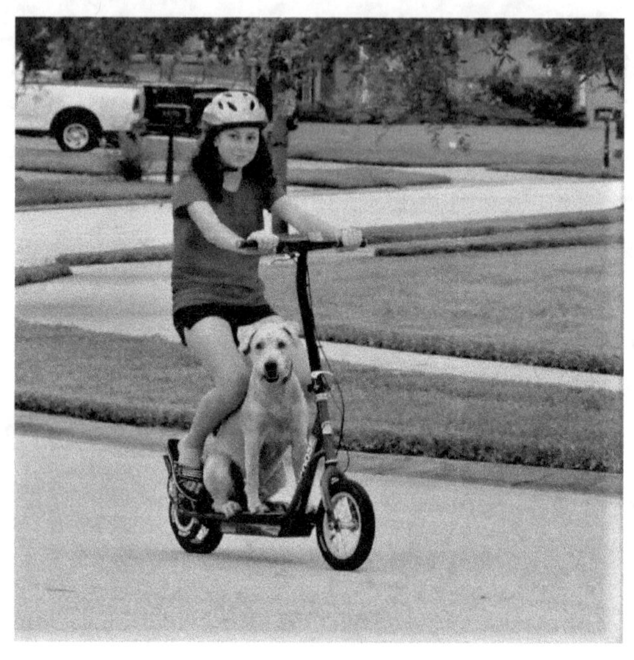

world.

Even with the small area that he had to sit on this motorized scooter, to trust her, and stay on it for such a long time was incredible!

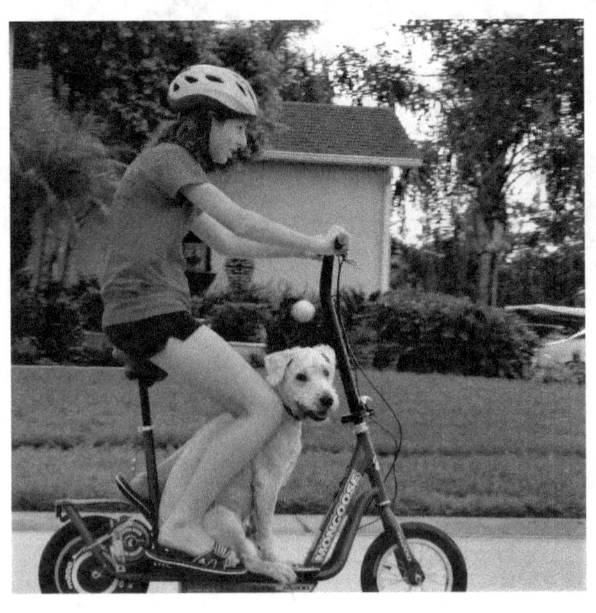

Such a personality! To smile at me as
they

we're going by with not a worry in the
world!

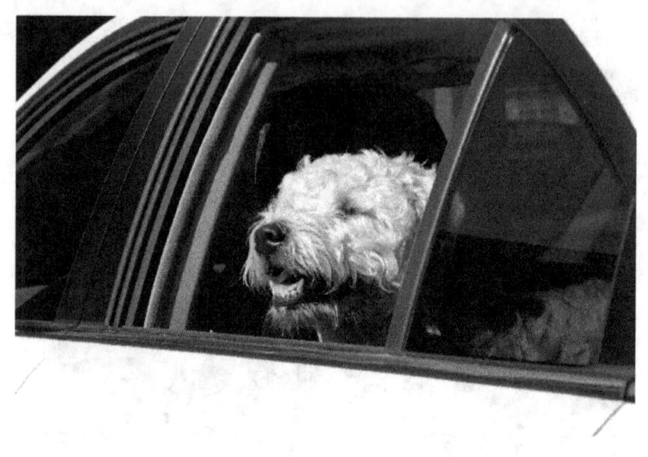

Buddy loved to go places in the car.

I always took note, looking in the rearview
mirror to see if there would be a change in his
behavior when I headed in the direction of
the Barr Street Trailhead of the Little Big
Econ State Forest.

Especially when there are four other trailheads to this gorgeous forest. He always showed excitement, which told me that he

could sense where we were going, by the turns, settings, and smells along the way! He loved it because on this trailhead we always spent hours in the forest, because one gets caught up in the quaintness of the seven bridges that you cross over, with poetic tributaries and see a variety of scenes, terrain and wildlife.

Then, the last bridge, meant that Buddy would be slowly easing himself in the water and swimming in the river.

11

Road Trips

Buddy has gone so many places with me. Writing them down, I find myself at awe. I drove him to New York City, in Queens, to visit relatives, and the first humorous event that comes to mind was when we were crossing the Washington Bridge approaching

Brooklyn, New York, Buddy was sitting shot gun, standing with his front paws on the door arm rest with his head out

the window, and nose stretched
straight up in the air, as if he were

smelling wondrous smells. The scene
of old worn dungeon apartments was
alarming, but Buddy lightened the
mood, as usual.

The next thing that happened was that
the traffic on the bridge came to a halt.
An accident I suppose. And then we
were noticed by an old black Cadillac,
filled with big guys that looked like
something out of the Goodfellas movie.
They all looked at us with big smiles
laughing, when they saw Buddy with
his nose up in the air and especially
when they noticed that our auto plate
showed that we were from Florida.
Buddy and I even got to walk through

Queens, N.Y. to a dog park and met
and spoke to the Queens New York
local dog owners.

 Buddy always made me feel
comfortable, relaxed, fun, any place
that I went with him. He also was
surprisingly agreeable with the
Queens, New Yorker Dogs too!

From there we went camping at a state
park in Connecticut, where in the
morning we watched fisherman
standing in the foggy/misty streams fly
fishing for a trout competition.

 Again, Buddy helped me to feel
accepted, and open for exploring
anywhere!

We also got to explore an old church,
which was converted into an Artist

Glass Blowing Studio and the real
chairs from the TV. Show

called Alfred Hitchcock Show, that I
used to watch as a child, along with
many other memorabilia.

The Artist was going to make some
awesome beveled colored glass
windows for a tree House that I was
planning on building on Clear
Landing, in Christmas, Florida.

Buddy was so well behaved.

Not far from the campground, was a
Drive-in Theatre. So, I thought that it
would be a fun memorable experience
of going to a Drive-in, so, Buddy and I
set out to go.

It seemed silly to go to a Drive-in with just my dog but there was nothing else to do so why not.

Of course, I stopped and got us both special foods to eat and snacks for entertainment. We arrived early and waited outside the gate on the side of a country road, and then it poured down rain, and they were going to cancel the movie. It stopped and they let us in, but we were the ONLY ones in the whole Drive-In Theatre!

Now what movie do you think was playing? Fortunately, I had not seen this movie before;

"Get Smart" a movie version taken from the TV. Show that I use to watch as a child! It was very humorous, and Buddy seemed to enjoy it too.

I wish that someone would have taken a photo of Buddy and me watching this movie, because we were both watching intensely. Yes, he was sitting up straight, shot gun and both of us enjoying the movie with our snacks!

We were on our way to stay at my artist friend Renee Lammers, who was living in Bar Harbor park, Maine, in a brand-new state of the art Air Streamer, with her husband and two large Golden Retrievers, named Daisy & Duke, that Buddy knew well, because she use to live in our neighborhood in Florida.

We went out and about, every day to

paint for hours, and the first time that
we left, we had to leave

Buddy with her dogs in her brand new,
state of the art, Air-Streamer, for
hours. When we came back, her place
looked like a gang of teenager's rams
shacked the place. Everything was
everywhere! But the dogs all appeared
happy and content.

There were some other camping, at
two different New England states that
we had to sleep in the car, in the
summer, with the windows up enough
so that no hands could reach in, while
we were sleeping, and it became hot
and miserable, and us both having to
adjust throughput the night.

What a real trooper of a dog! He also
scoped out a porcupine!

I even found myself and Buddy
camping in St. Augustine, Amelia
Island, and others near Micanopy,
Florida, so that Loren could go to a
Horse Summer Camp, in case
something happened, I would be
nearby, so Buddy and I

went everywhere. He always was a
good sport! Another time I took him
camping with me to St. Augustine, he
walked with me and looked at all the
Artwork and he patiently waited while
I spent time talking to the many
artists.

It was cold and he sat with me while I

made a campfire and sat talking to my
sister on the phone.

Then I remember it being very cold
and we snuggled up in my sleeping
bag, in our tent, to keep each other
warm.

I've even taken Buddy a couple of
times to the Wild Horse Rescue
Center, in Mims, Florida, where I had
rescued my horse, Homer, which had
29 Wild Mustangs, a gorgeous stallion,

named Romeo, Ponies, 5 Dogs, Pigs,
Ducks, and Chickens.

The owner said don't worry about it. If
he misbehaves, to discipline him, and
to let him that know that you mean it!

So, I let my guard down, relaxed and
let him go.

The next thing that I noticed was that
Buddy was going into all the Wild
Mustang horses' stalls, barking and
charging them. One kicked him and he
left. Just when I thought everything
was good, I saw him with a chicken's
head completely in his mouth!

Buddy was like a wild kid in a candy
store, and Luckily, he did not get hurt.

12

Natural Instinct's

It has always surprised me when Buddy displayed natural instincts, when it came to other animals.

He knew better to not attack an alligator!

One very hot summer day while I was

in the cabin, at my place I named Clear
Landing, in Christmas, Florida, while
on my cell phone, I saw something out

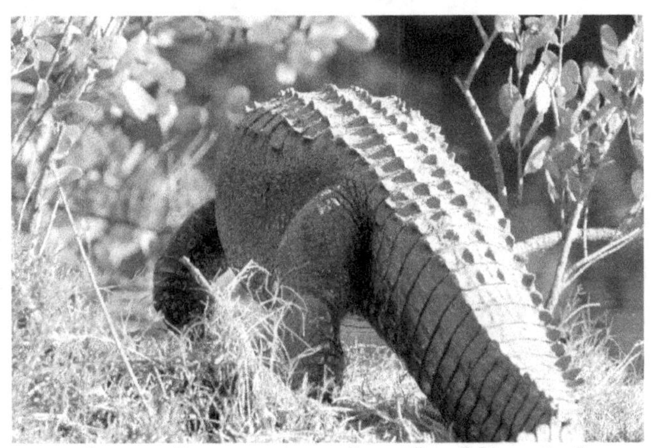

by my large over a hundred live Oak
Tree, which looked like a snake. The
grass was high, so it was unclear what
it might be. When I went out to get a
better look, I could see that it was an
alligator!

I thought that it was strange that my soft- Coated Wheaton Terrier dog, Captain Buddy, who was only about eight feet away lying

under the wraparound deck did not bark or come charging out like he usually does immediately, when he sees a squirrel. An instinct, I suppose.

I quickly got him in the cabin. The Alligator now was in front of my car, faced with his tail back to me. I knew that an alligator can run about 40 mph, so I thought that I would just stand behind him and watch him runaway. To my surprise, the alligator abruptly turned around, looked me square in the eyes ready to attack me! We just stared at each other, which

seemed like a long time. I could see
that his eyes were a real pale green, in
the hot summer sun, but

it was my eyes that were wide open as I
stood frozen, staring at the alligator,
not knowing what to do next!

I made a dash to get in my car. I
quickly turned my key in the ignition,
and hit the gas to run over this gator,
but my tires didn't hit him. I drove
around and around on my circle drive,
but I never saw him again.

Buddy has also shown natural instincts
to being cautious to in our subdivision
when there would be the tall Sandhill

cranes in front of us or alongside of the
sidewalk, he never attempted to charge
or attack them like he would a rabbit
or a duck.

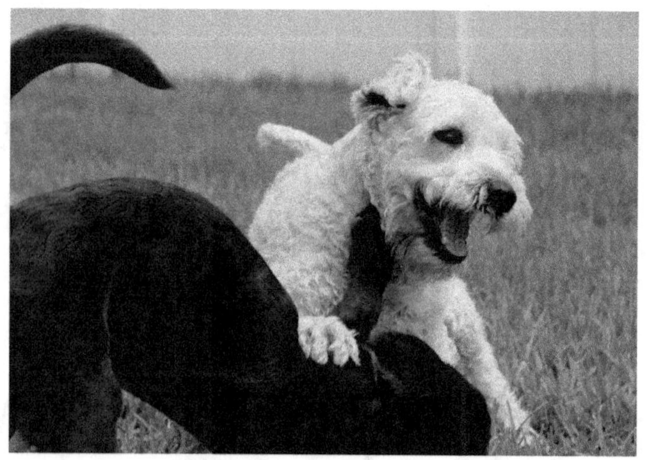

13

Buddy's Dog Friends

Is there anything purer than seeing
dogs running around and chasing each
other's tails? Seeing dogs having fun
makes pretty much everyone smile.

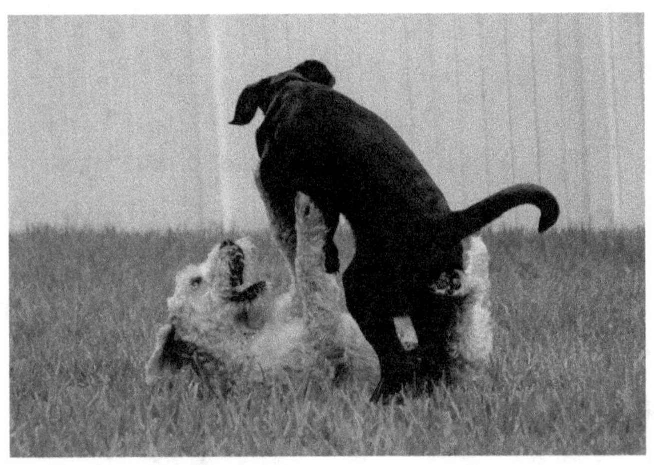

This is the first one of

Captain Buddy wrestling with his Black

Labrador friend named DJ.

Taking Buddy to the many different
dog parks, helped me to enjoy the
simple pleasures in life, seeing him
happy, meeting other dogs and making
new friends made it all worth it.

This was Buddies Birthday, that I was
able to get another Wheaton to play with

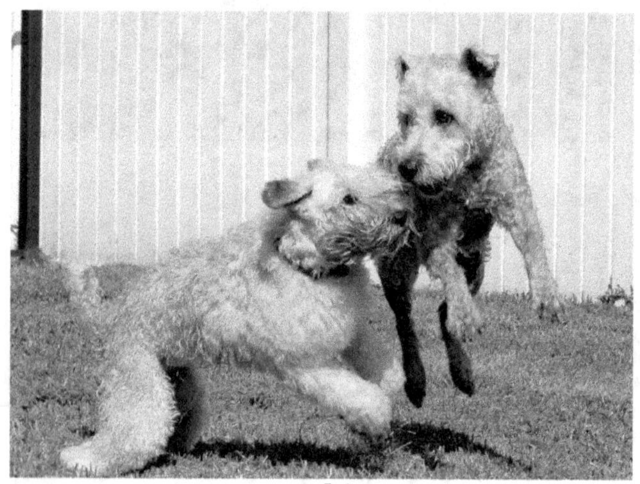

him.

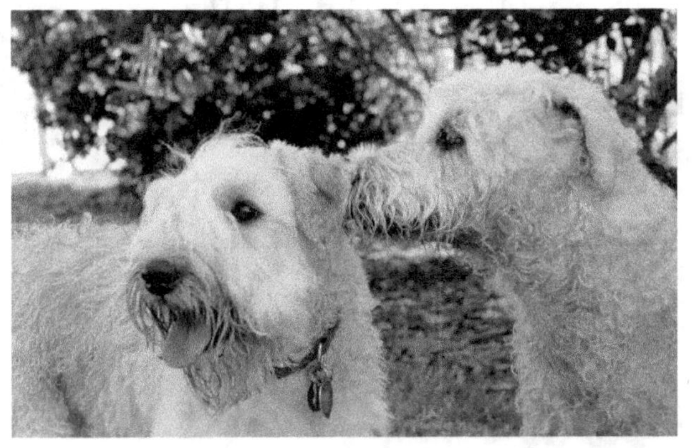

As you can see that Buddy is wet and Annie is

not!

This is another Wheaton Terrier

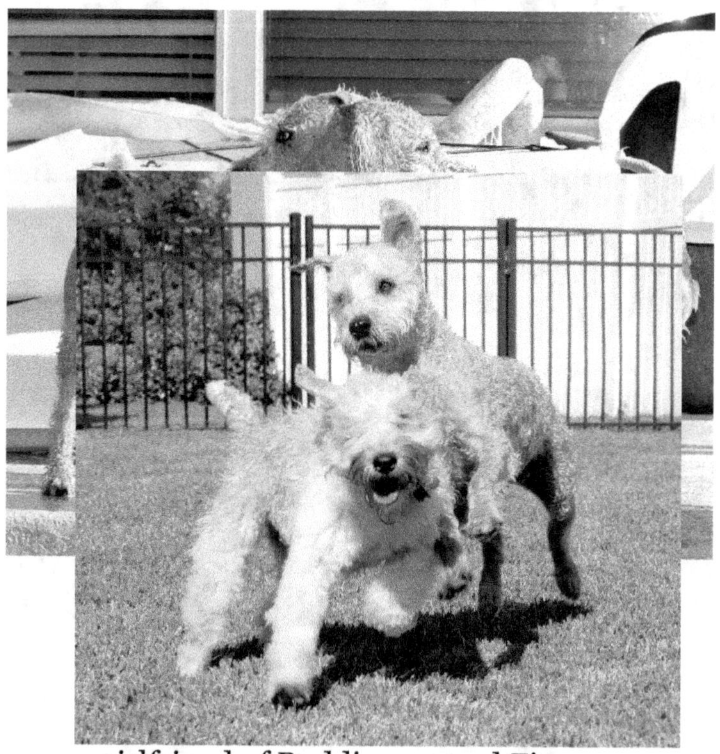

girlfriend of Buddies, named Ziggy.

She was Buddy's first encounter with another Wheaton, that we met at the Riverside Dog Park. Her owner

brought Ziggy over to our house to swim in the pool. They quietly just stared at each other, did not make a sound, and then slowly they locked necks together.

It was very emotionally moving!

The next time that Buddy saw her at the park, he was so focus on playing with her, that when another dog came up behind him and intervened, Buddy immediately attacked him.

I guess that he was jealous or was protecting her.

14

Intelligence

Buddy was very intelligent!

I don't know where to begin. It's not
just about doing tricks, it's about
Buddy knowing how each of us felt or
the place where we were coming from,
that he seemed to be so in tuned with

knowing what was going on by

sensing our emotions.

In this pic Loren had moved out of the
house, was only visiting, and she was
living with her boyfriend, who owned a
dog, named Boomer. When she would

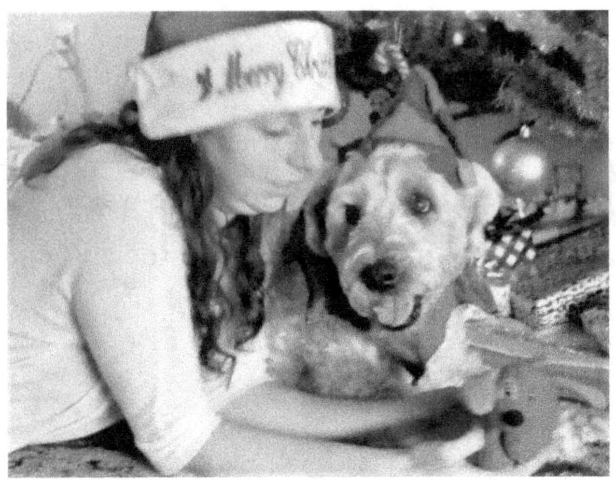

come over with Boomer, Buddy and
him never really played with each
other like Buddy did with his other dog
friends. He seemed to shut down, or

not be as open and expressive.

This Christmas day, she came over alone and was spending some original quality time with

him. You can tell that he was really soaking up Loren's attention, even though she wasn't playing with him, just her presence was all that he needed at this time in his life.

This is another time that I was able to capture
Buddy showing empathy and concern.

This was the first time that Loren is

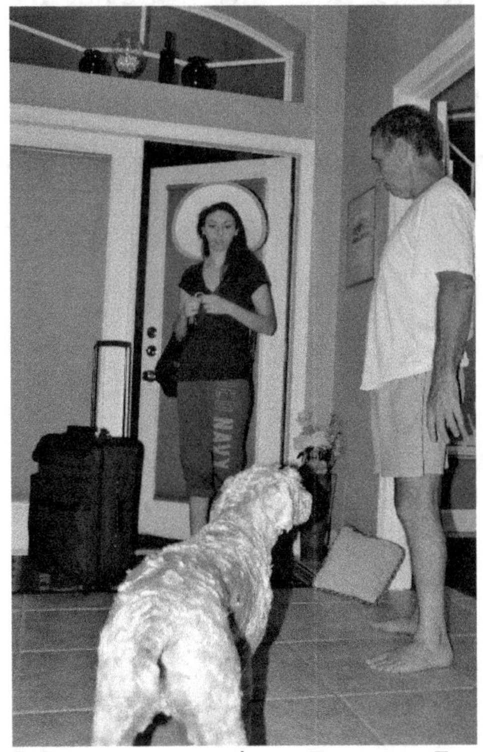

going away on a trip to Daytona Beach,

College Spring Break, to stay in a
Hotel, on the Beach, to spend some
time with all her girlfriends.

  You can tell from Buddy's
gestures/emotions of concerns
through that of Loren's Dad. You can
tell that her Dad's fingers are not in a
relaxed gesture, which shows he is
understandably concerned, and Buddy
is picking up on that emotion and his
aura.

Here is Buddy, going to bury and hide
this huge bone, which I would give to
him for long cold winter days, when all
of us were at work/school.

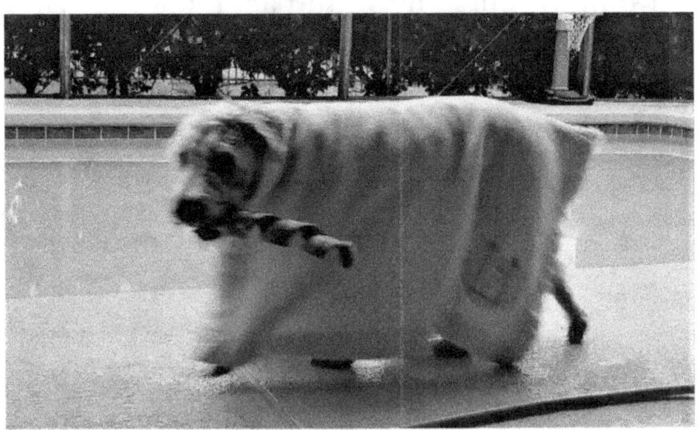

He would save some for as long as
multiple weeks, and then go and dig
them up, remembering where he
buried them.

I caught him in the act of going to bury
this huge rawhide!

Also, when I would walk Buddy in our

 subdivision and we would go by a
rabbit or duck, he would act like he
wasn't going to do anything even
though he would be looking right at
them all the while we were going by,
but just after he past them, he would
then bolt out at them!

Captain Richard

&

Captain Buddy

Ironically, the last four years of
Buddy's life

was spent mostly with Richard.

Yes, the one that was so adamant
about not getting a dog in the first
place.

He started working from home, and so
he spent all day with Buddy.

This really put a twist on Richard being more empathetic with Buddy.

It would be noticed time after time how Buddy would bow down to Richard and listen to his commands and look at him with eager attention.

I remember reading once that Dogs have an instinct to view the male of the household as the alpha!

For example; he walked Buddy without a leash, and Buddy would listen to the slightest little sound or even just a gesture, from Richard to stop, sit, and wait up ahead at an intersection in our subdivision, before crossing.

Buddy even got to go with Richard when he had to do errands. The errands were mostly to Home Depot, or Lowe's, where Buddy was commanded to hop from his truck onto

the low riding steel carts. Buddy sat
straight up, with a smile on his face,
sitting still as can be and it always
amazed everyone, from customers to
employees, on how well Buddy
behaved!

Buddy and Richard would go to the
Riverside Park/Dog Park, without on a
leash, and Buddy would follow his
commands. Richard would also walk
Buddy down to the Tennis Courts, in
our subdivision, where there is a lake,
and they would sit under a Live Oak
tree together. Richard said, that after
about twenty minutes, Buddy would
just stand up and look at him as if to
say, well it's time to go.

Then Richard would get up and they
would walk home.

Buddy also became an icon, lying at
the floor of Richards's computer chair,

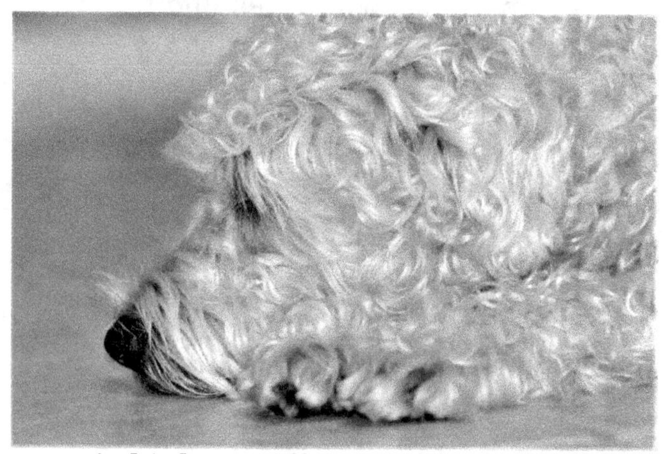

in his home office, while he worked.

It was as if he knew that this area was

important, and he was dedicated to
doing his

part as an FAA agent!

Part Two:

After Thoughts

The

Benefits of Owning

a Dog

1

Live life to its fullest!

To live life to the fullest means facing your fears with heroism, an open mind, and a lack of prejudice. It means making the most of what you have and never settling for less than the life you are capable of living. It means being truly alive and awake to life and not asleep in life's waiting room.

The first day, waking up, after Buddy's death, I remember feeling his absence by realizing that I was immediately thinking of seeing him, to lift my spirits, in just looking at his hopeful face, his instant energy and realizing very quickly on how much I looked for life through his eyes and positive moves. He was always full of life, no matter what. He never gave up on me.

He never gave a hesitant look or cautionary gestures. He sometimes on a Saturday, would be waiting for as long as five hours for me to be able to take him out and about. And when I finally did, even though he would be sound asleep, after following me all around the house attending to chores, he would quickly jump up on all fours and be wagging his tail, ahead of me with a big smile on his face, glee in his eyes and a bounce in his walk, not showing any disappointment of any kind.

When he left, the first message to me was live life to the fullest!

He always perked up with a bounce in his walk when entering a forest. Even when he was sick, he displayed a stronger urge to go into Tosohatchee, (33,000 acres of forest), but I didn't have the time. I still can't get over that he didn't even display any pain, even though the Veterinarian said that he had cancer of the stomach.

He stuck it out to the very end.

It seemed as if he was taking note of each one of us that came to his bed side the last days of his death, to sense that we were ok. Meaning, that even though he had been lying in his bed for days, without being able to get any more water down him, he would open his eyes when talking to him Even the last week of having a stomach tumor, he greeted me at the door or came running to greet me, coming home from work, as I was getting out of the car.

What an astounding devoted dog! Before him being sick, coming home later than usual and going to the back, sliding glass door you would be greeted with a dog so happy to see you that he would be jumping straight high up into the air with his head going about five feet high!

<u>I never realized how much I thought about Buddy until he was gone.</u>

As soon as I walk in the house, for a split second, I think Buddy is coming to greet me, or where's Buddy's smiling face and wagging tail to lift my spirits? He/a Dog becomes an extension of one's self in so many ways.

He enhanced my life, physically, mentally, spiritually and made me a better person. He gave me more confidence and was very empathetic.

Apart of me thinks it to be cruel to just own one dog. Buddy was in most part alone and didn't get to play much with other dogs, because of his terrier territorial characteristics, and there

were very few dogs that he could play
with, so I always wished that he had
another dog to play with.

I remember when we did find a dog
that he got along with and the dog
didn't want to go in the water, Buddy
would have a fit and would get real,
aggravated with the dog because they
didn't like the water too. But then
again, I think that you should have just
one dog because you are his buddy.

I think that this is what is keeping me
from getting another dog. Also,
because I keep trying to see Buddy in
each dog that I look at, and then I tell
myself, that there will never be another
dog like Buddy! It is probably going to
take some time for me to get over
Buddy.

2

Unconditional

Love & Devotion

To define unconditional love is to say
that a person loves someone
unselfishly, that he or she cares about
the happiness of the other person and
will do anything to help that person
feel happiness without expecting
anything in return. In other words, the
definition of unconditional love is
"love without

conditions."

I can totally say all these things with only

 Buddy in mind, but never of any person.

Unconditional love is easy; no decision- making or responsibility is required. Love has no boundaries when it's unconditional. But the real world is conditional. There are reactions to actions and consequences, too. Each of us has at least one marital condition in mind; fidelity, honesty, loyalty, and truth.

Unconditional love is a love that lasts and persists despite any sort of negativity toward the one giving the love. The root of

unconditional love is understanding
and forgiveness. The greatest and
ultimate example of this type of love is
Jesus Christ.

It may seem silly to think of a dog
being devoted, but it is real, and it
gives one confidence in setting out to
doing something just knowing that
something alive is going with you
whole heartedly without any
hesitation, or resentment.

It's this feeling of

total devotion, that gives you inner
strength, makes you feel free, positive
and strong about what you are setting
out to do. Buddy's personality was so
real. I believe that the more one on one

that you spend with your dog, the
more empathy will be applied, and the
more emotionally you will feel towards
your dog.

3

To See Life Through That of

a

Child, Everything Is New

Kids are fascinated by everything because it's all new to them. Every day is new to them, so everything seems exciting and full of possibilities.

This is how it felt being around Buddy. You don't know what to expect. You find yourself being more observant of your surroundings and he was always

unpredictable, full of energy, life and

everything was new to him, so I would
find myself clicking into that mindset
just being around him and watching
his reactions to his surroundings.
Doing this helped me to be more
observant of my surroundings and

people in them.

Everything Is a Learning Experience

Children are interested in learning as
much as they can.

They want to know everything!

Walking Buddy I saw things that I
wouldn't see if he was not with me.

He made me really appreciate my surroundings. Whether it be an animal in the forest near us, a dog across the four lanes of our main street in our subdivision, or a rabbit, deer, duck, armadillo, Opossum, in our back yard.

Just as in art, drawing is all about seeing, and the more we see the more we know, and the more we know the richer our life will be.

Buddy helped make my life richer.

4

Everyone Is a Possible Friend

Studies show that just looking at a dog, will help you to let down your guard.

Therefore, many of TV. Commercials have animals, mostly dogs, in them, because it is a way for them to help open your mind and take an open-minded approach to their product and their way of thinking. People are more open minded, and more

likely will communicate with someone
with a dog.

Children are always open to meeting
new people. They want to smile and
make friends and learn people's names
and what they do and why.

I would find myself more likely to talk
to strangers when I would have Buddy
with me. It was either, because after
they would show an openness,
appreciation through his looks, or
excellent behavior, it would help me to
let down my guard, smile back and be
more open-minded, understanding,
and appreciative of them.

Or it would also be because if they had
a dog also, such as while walking in our
neighborhood, I would take time to

talk, so that Buddy would have the enjoyment of meeting another dog.

So, this constant open-minded attitude, helped create a stronger bond for us as well as keeping each other happy!

The best part of being a kid, is not spending time worrying about what people think, but to be more focused on you, who you are, to capture your own spirit, to feel more confident and proud to feel free to do what you want to do.

Imagine how free you'd feel if you didn't care what people thought about you? Not to the extent to totally let yourself go, or become the office eccentric person, but just enough so

that you do things you want to do
without worrying what others will
think.

I would experience total strangers to
be more open-minded and excepting of
me through seeing the cuteness of
Buddy, or the mannerisms that he
displayed, in turn this allowed me to
do or feel the way I wanted to.

5

World Full of Possibilities

Like children, Buddy was in most part positive in attitude, always eager to try something new, especially if it's presented to him as an adventure. Buddy made things feel like a game so you're not wasting time and energy moping around, dreading what comes next. He made life feel simple, easy and fun.

We shouldn't limit ourselves to what seems right or practical, when we can think like a child and do what we really want.

Being around Buddy helped me to think that I could do what I wanted to, within limits of course, but I would take him places that helped me to think outside the box and not worry what others thought.

Being around Buddy gave me that feeling that anything is possible, with his positive attitude and he was so unpredictable. This goes hand in hand with thinking that the world is full of possibilities and you can get in on any of them.

A positive attitude always opens others minds and helps you to be successful in life.

It can be very refreshing, when I experienced this through my students in my art classroom.

Being around Buddy, gave me the mindset to take the time to just let my mind wonder. To slow my pace and observe the simplicity of the lines, shapes, textures, forms, values, and colors of objects as I walked him. The tasks will still be there when you're ready to get to them. I always said, one should take the time to smell the roses.

6

Your Imagination Is Limitless

Being an Art Teacher, helped me to use my imaginations limitless, as a child. a child doesn't care what's real and what could happen because they want it to, so in their mind, it's so.

They can remove the barriers on logical thinking.

Once your imagination can roam more

freely, you can use it to tackle home
and work tasks and it helped me to see
how innovative improved, because of
taking the time to use my imagination.

I know that because of owning Buddy,
and spending a lot of time with him,
gave me that carefree feeling as a child,
which helped me to be more
imaginative in my everyday

thinking.

7

Give one inspiration to

go on in life

Inspire means to excite, encourage, or breathe life into. Inspire comes from the Latin word that means to inflame or to blow in to. When you inspire something, it is as if you are blowing air over a low flame to make it grow.

A film can be inspired by a true story.

Captain Buddy made me feel so happy

about the simplest things, it was like
being in a movie.

A true story but a lively one!

Inspiration awakens us to new
possibilities by allowing us to
transcend our ordinary experiences
and limitations.

Inspiration propels a person from
apathy to possibility and transforms
the way we perceive our own
capabilities. Inspiration may
sometimes be overlooked because of
its elusive nature.

8

Caregiver Response

A dog's face features trigger caregiver response. They're called social releasers it triggers in an innate caregiver response in humans.

Buddy kept me wanting to care for him until the very end.

Every morning, I made sure to clean his face, that the water was warm, on a fresh washcloth, cleared his eyes of gunk, washed his nose, brushed his teeth, massaged his gums, brushed his

coat, would clean and put ear drops
and massage his ears.

In purpose, we find energy. In energy,
we find creativity, productivity, and
engagement.

Meaning making makes meaningful
lives.

This one sentence is so powerful.

We all need a purpose in life in order
to drive us forward with confidence.
Just taking Buddy for a walk, gave me
energy and helped keep me in shape.
Knowing that I am satisfying his needs,
helped me to appreciate myself, be
more confident, empathetic and in
turn appreciate others and have more
energy to help others, thus making my

life richer because of that extra energy,
that Buddy initially gave me each

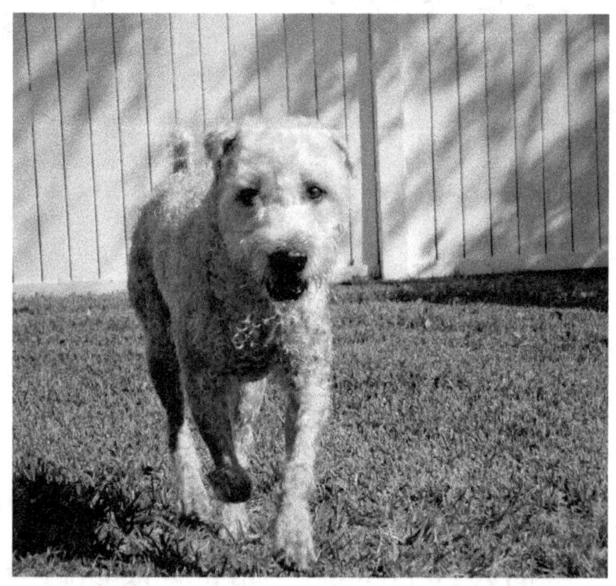

morning before going to work and in
the evening as well.

9

The Simplest Things in Life

Some things in life fill us with joy even though they are such small, simple things.

They provide moments of pure magic that bring us back into the present moment and make us grateful for everything we have in life.

Here are such little pleasures that we should all seek to enjoy more often.

Getting up early, while taking Buddy
for a walk, pretending that I am him,

watching the back of his head, as he
led the way, and focusing on the subtle
turn of his ears to guide my eyes and
thoughts up ahead, made it even more
enjoyable.

Giving Buddy a big Hug helped me to
want to hug someone else.

There are chemicals released, called,
Oxytocin, which also is expressed as
the love hormone, when we hug those
we love.

Standing at one end of my pool, on a
hot summer day, counting out 1, while
bringing my hands up in the air, then
putting them both behind me,
counting out 2, always brought out a

cry and bark in Buddy, while jumping
and running around the pool, excited
to know that I am about to jump in,

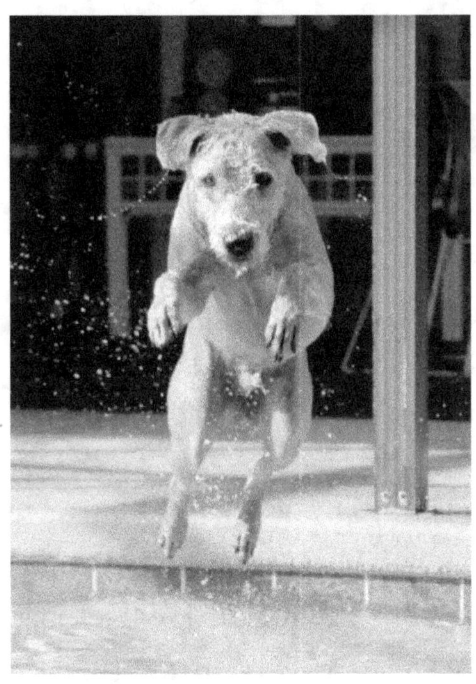

only to wait for me to bring both
hands forward say 3, and then jump in
the cool water after me!

Ice cream on a hot day, when you are melting in the heat, grab an ice cream and experience immediate happiness. Whatever flavour you go for, you'll be left feeling happy and full of pleasure and a lot cooler!

It was not only enjoyable for me, but giving Buddy his Dog Ice Cream, and watch him lick it, one lick at a time, and then to lick the rim of his bowl, round and around, multiple times, without lifting his tongue once, ameliorated to emphasize my feelings as well.

It always seemed that Buddy was
talking to me with his facial
expressions.

Scientists have discovered that dogs

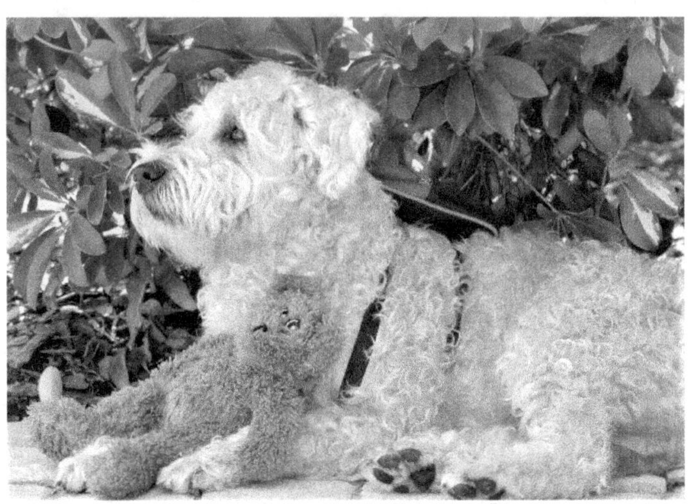

can voluntarily use their

facial expressions of communication.

So much of animal behavior is uncertain that the possibilities of a dog

seeing something a human can't, is not out of the question.

Finding shade on a sunny day while walking Buddy, he would stop sometimes and look up at me with his golden-brown eyes, black eyelashes, and white fluffy eyebrows/Ferrell and I would then find a nice shady spot under a tree or bench overlooking a lake in our subdivision, or the river in the Econ State Forest to relax.

Spontaneous events are just what we need. Whether you're a planner or just

like sticking to your routine,
spontaneity is a simple pleasure in life
that deserves a lot more attention!

Buddy was always ready when I was
ready.

The first dip in the pool/lake is a
refreshing feeling and always fun to see
Buddy's reaction, when I decided to
take a plunge in the pool. I would first
stand at the far end of the pool, stick my
big toe to test the temperature, Buddy
would let out a bark, jump forward with
all fours, and standing at the pool side,
be looking at me with anticipations.
After diving in, listening to if he dove in
as well!

It then was fun to swim up and gently
grab one of his cute soft chucky paws
and hold him for a second so that I

would beat him to the other end of the pool. His reaction was so cute, because he would whine, and bark more letting me know that I cheated!

Sitting around a cosy campfire, with friends and family, is another simple enjoyment in life, engaging, warm, and refreshing.

When I couldn't be with friends around a campfire, I could still enjoy it with Buddy, and talk to my friends on the phone.

Making someone smile is one of the simplest pleasures in life, and one of the easiest things to do. The feeling you get when you realize you've cheered someone up is brilliant. Even though Buddy was just a dog, he did look like he was smiling and when I saw him smiling it made me smile and if we were around other people, friends or strangers, we brought smiles to them as well!

Cooking breakfast on a Saturday morning were great for fixing a special breakfast for myself and Buddy.

He loved bacon and eggs easy over, especially when the eggs came from our own chickens on our farm, where Buddy managed to get one of my chickens, jumping out of the car window, when parked at the farm.

Cooking your favourite dish is so much fun, then afterwards, watching Captain Buddy, show his appreciation, by

taking his tongue ever so slowly
around the rim of his dog dish!

Especially after a Thanksgiving Feast!

10

Health Benefits

Owning a dog, reduces stress, blood pressure,
lowers heart rate, slows breathing, relaxes
muscle tension, in reduces depression. Talk to
a stranger or at least create a smile. Studies
show that a simple positive interaction with a
stranger will make us happier.

Some dogs can detect cancer, they can let diabetics know when their blood sugar is low.

This always made me wonder how much buddy or any dog was aware of human's feelings or emotions scientists are using

methods to decode animal behaviors.

Everyone needs to be seen, heard, and valued in life. Knowing that someone you care about wants to make plans to spend more time with you always feels great. Making plans is a good way to feel important and involved, which explains why it's a simple joy in life.

It may seem silly, but it's true that Captain Buddy, knew when I was taking him somewhere special!

I used sign language such as if we were
leaving exceptionally early to spend long
hours in the forest, I would place my
forefinger to my lips, to be quiet, pat my rear
end, for him to follow and he would quickly
and quietly be right behind me all the way!

 I did this for many years.

Being outside in the fresh air is good for us,
both physically and mentally. Studies show
that relationships grow stronger when spent
outdoors. Without the confines of indoor
walls, nature helps us to be ourselves and be
more open-minded, thus letting down our
guard, communicating and sharing more.

Being outdoors helps us to escape the stresses
in our lives and have a full refresh outlook on
life. If it we're not for Buddy,

 I would not have gone in the forest alone. He

helped me to be able to explore and experience some sense of adventure in my life. Since Buddy's death, I find myself having the urge to want to go outside, to get some fresh air, as if my body became conditioned to

going out more for fresh air, because I was outside more times when Buddy was alive. Especially, before going to bed at night, I would walk outside with him so that he could relieve himself for a good night's sleep.

I find myself still doing this, and I find that it gives me a more restful sleep as well.

Giving Buddy a shower or bath after a long

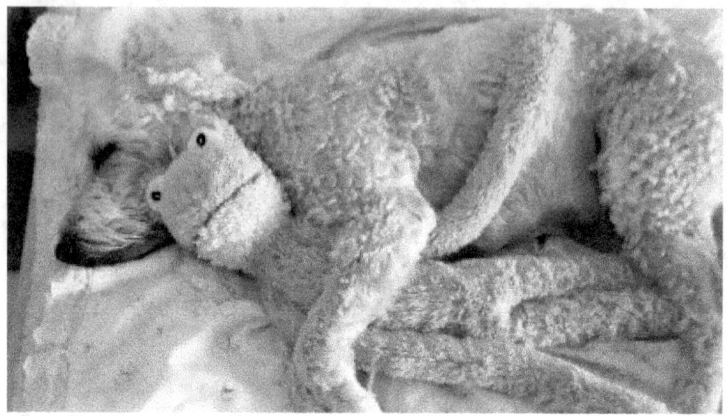

day instantly relieves stress.

Laughing with a good friend, or Captain Buddy, helped me to relieve stress, and enjoy life. Enjoying an afternoon nap, or laying out on the lounge by the pool, with Buddy, with a full moon gentle spring breeze, gave me soft comforting feelings.

Sitting on the beach, listening to the ocean or in the forest.

Being with Buddy was always inviting to just sit down and take in all the sounds of nature. Such as the soothing ocean sounds or that of nature, helped slow my mind down and let me drift off into a chilled place.

 Listening to ocean waves and sounds in the forest is such a great way to connect with nature too.

Having some alone time after a busy day, is so good for your mind and body, making it one of the best, easiest pleasures in life.

It was easy having alone time with Buddy, especially when we were in the forest. Knowing that no one was around, surrounded by nature, and knowing that he would protect me,

really helped me to think things
through in life.

When your pet choosing to sit with
you, it gives you a huge rush of joy.
Especially when they rest their head on
your leg. Having a pet, you love to
want to spend time with you and be
close to you is one of the best feelings
in the world.

Buddy loved to lay with me, either on
the hammock swing, at the pool side or
in my bed, while I read, watched TV. or
camping in a tent or at the cabin, I
named Clear Landing, in Christmas,
Florida.

Finishing work early is so satisfying to
get back to enjoying your downtime or

hobbies.

It means that you've got everything done and you can sit back and relax.

Coming home early, to see Buddy light up, smiling, jumping up in the air, as tall as me, feeling his supper soft coat, and giving him a big hug, was also very gratifying.

Spending time outdoors with Buddy always was a great workout. It really boosted his spirits, and in turn, he made it easier for me to give energy.

This is Buddy on the Barr Street
Trailhead, in the Little Big Econ State

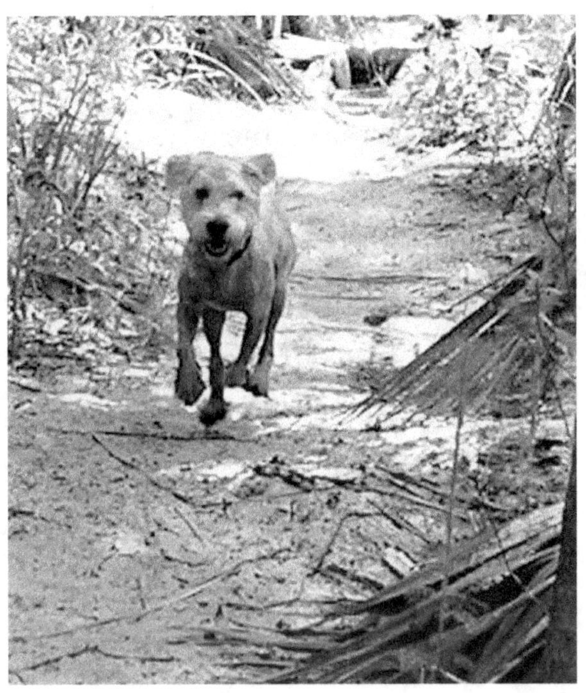

Forest, (10,000 acres of forest), where
you go over seven different quaint
wooden bridges, over tributaries of the

Econlockhatcee River, on a five-mile
round trip, and we didn't just hike this
trail, we would be doing something
else along the way.

Either sitting on the riverbank while I

sketched, painted, photographed or
observed alligators, Bald Eagles,
canoeists, deer, raccoon, fish,
armadillo, etc.

I always found myself to be drawn into
the forest, not realizing how far or how
long we were in the forest, because
Buddy always made me feel like a kid,
with endless energy!

11

Teaches Responsibility

Being responsible: makes one's life richer. When you do what you have promised, people see you as a responsible and reliable person.

Which in return gives you more self-esteem and self-worth. Personal responsibility is taking ownership of your actions.

Buddy helped me to be more

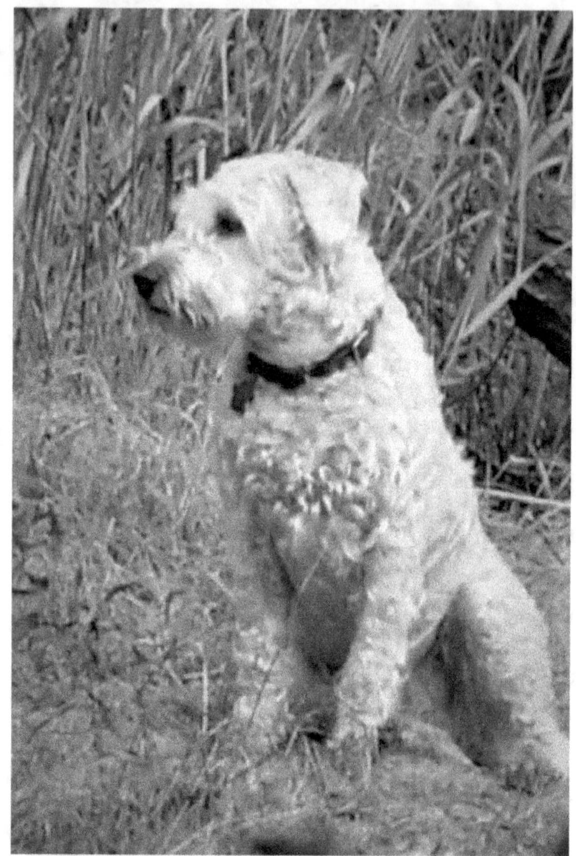

responsible, because being with Buddy

made me happy, and more

appreciative of everything and

everyone, so I wanted to be the best that I could. It seems silly, but it's true. Think about it, just being around a soft, white, fluffy, cute, energetic, sweet, and unstoppable with dedication of unconditional love, makes it so easy to be responsible!

Place others' needs before your own is being responsible and being consistent.

Being reliable shows people can depend on you to do what you say you're going to do.

When you have things to look forward to in your own life, like having a dog, like Buddy, you will more likely want to make other people's lives more enjoyable.

Holding yourself accountable for your actions, means that when you do something wrong, own up to it. It may seem silly, but when you know that you have a strong, reliable dog in your life, it makes you a stronger person, and when you feel strong inside, you are more apt to admit when you are wrong.

Tell the truth to keep your relationships authentic. Try to be as honest as you can, as honesty shows you are responsible enough to tell the truth.

Keep in touch with loved ones and friends. Show you are actively trying to spend time with them.

Try to figure out how you can do better. Think before you speak to show you care and take time to think your words through.

Learn to think about other people's thoughts and feelings.

Empathy is viewing other's feelings from their perspectives, what it would feel like, if it were you. When you say something or do something, think about how it will make the other person feel.

Being responsible is not putting off your tasks until after you've had fun. Start by doing what you need to get done first, so that you can relax and have fun.

12

Feeling Loved Every Day

Having a positive outlook, means allowing your happiness to shape your present as well as your future. Buddy helped me to feel love every day. I think that it was mostly his constant unconditional love that gave me strength to go on in life.

Many scientific studies show that a dog, can help someone live

longer. Especially, the elderly,
and those that raised a family and now
the kids have all moved out of their
parents' homes.

When you stare at your dog,
both your oxytocin levels go up, the
same as when you pet them and play
with them.

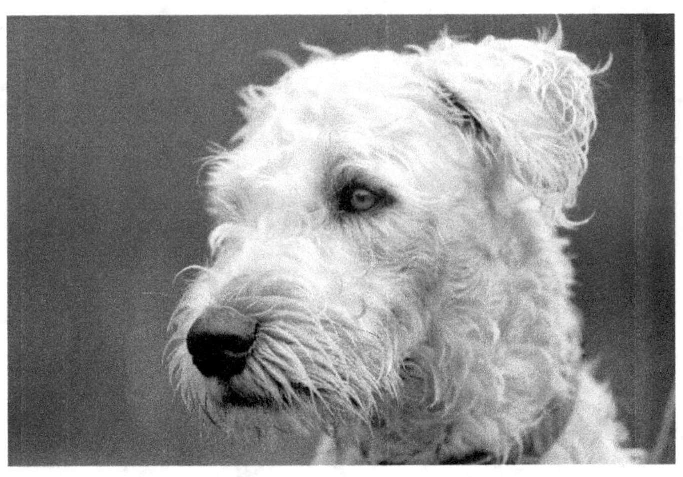

Coming home after a trip away, such as when I worked one summer in Yellowstone National Park, and upon my return, I found him sitting at the front glass door, same as when I had

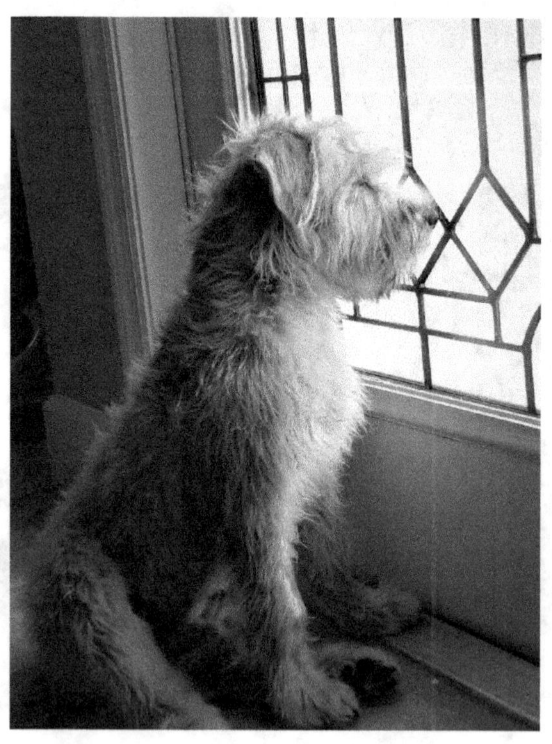

previously left him over a month before leaving.

My husband said that he was waiting there everyday, in anticipating of my return.

Just a little trivia about Yellowstone National Park, we camped in every campsite in Yellowstone, 2.4 million acres, and the only campsite that allowed dogs, was the Madison campsite. One thing that we noticed while camping at Madison, the dogs walked like they were show dogs, with a bounce in their gait, head up high and their nose up straight. When I ask the owners if they were show dogs, they said no that they never saw them walk like this either.

I think that it is because they could smell smells that they've never smelled before, such as there only ancestor, the Wolf.

I did this another summer for a month, when I went on a plein - air, painting workshops in Maine and to Monhegan Island, (10 miles, off the coast of Maine) Also, when I took my art students, to camp and volunteer their services to Yellowstone National Park, another summer, by painting picnic tables, famous gravestone fencing, parking lot, and gathering trash.

Coming home and knowing that Buddy would still show happiness, helped me to feel free, still loved, and to be able to explore on my own as well.

Another summer when I went out
West, 12 different states, 5,000 miles,
to see some relatives for the first time.
Buddy never gave me what's called the
standoff, like when my horse felt
betrayed.

I guess it has something to do with his
characteristics. Remember, when we
first went into the pet store to get a
dog, and I read the characteristics of
his breed, not being a clingy dog,
because they have their own
independence.

Reflecting on owning Captain Buddy, I selected some of my favorite, famous quotes about dogs that I know are so true.

<u>Here are some of my top picks;</u>

"A dog is the only thing on earth that loves you more than you love yourself."

"The best therapist has fur and four legs."

"One way to get the most out of life, is to look upon it as an Adventure."

"Dogs are not our whole life, but they make our lives whole".

"The world would be nicer place if everyone had the ability to love unconditionally as a dog."

"When I look into the eyes of an animal, I do not see an animal. I see a living being. I see a friend. I feel a soul."

"Until one has loved an animal, a part of one's soul remains unawaken."

"What a beautiful world it would be, if people had hearts like dogs."

"Bliss is the result of a silent conversation
between me and my dog."

"A dog can make you feel rich."

13

Most Paramount Dog

When we first got Buddy, I thought to myself, that we were going to have to really watch him, and take care of him, but Captain Buddy took great care of us as

well!

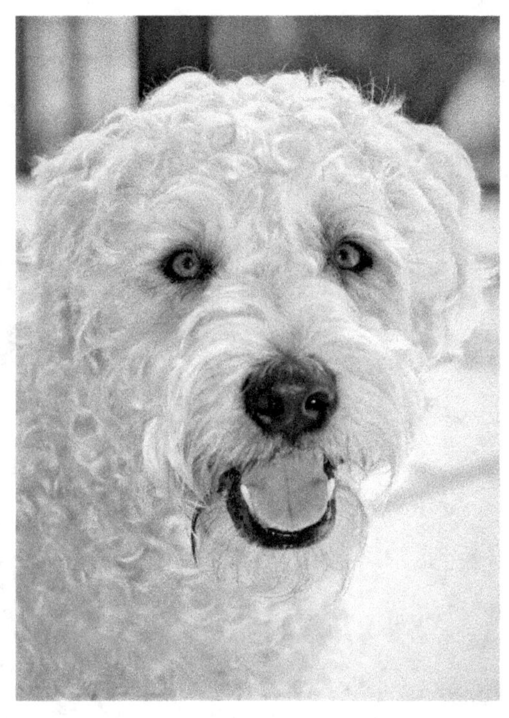

Dogs help keep their owners'

lives balanced;

Physically, Mentally,

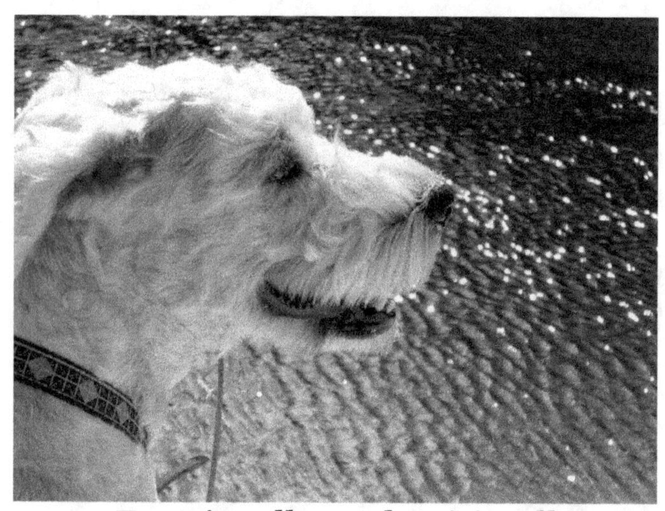

Emotionally, and Spiritually!

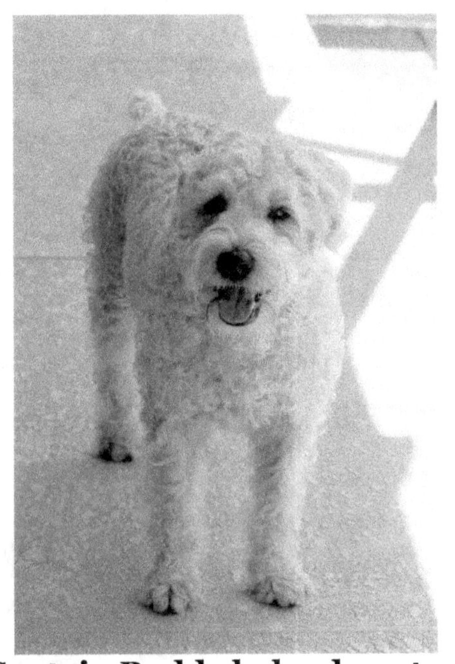

**Captain Buddy helped me to do
all the**

**things that I have shared with
you in this book.**

Specially to stand

my ground!

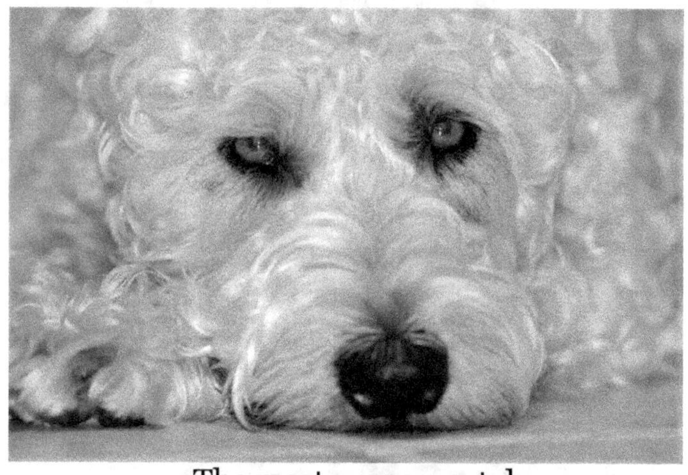

The most paramount dog
that I have ever owned!
The incredible, unstoppable
Captain Buddy!

A gift from the angels!

The End

www.ingramcontent.com/pod-product-compliance
Lightning Source LLC
Chambersburg PA
CBHW070802240726
48654CB00007B/173